The Science of rhBMP-2

THE SCIENCE OF rhBMP-2

William F. McKay, ME
Vice President
Biologics Research and Development
Medtronic Sofamor Danek, Inc.
Memphis, Tennessee

Steven M. Peckham, PhD
Manager
Biologics Research and Development
Medtronic Sofamor Danek, Inc.
Memphis, Tennessee

James S. Marotta, PhD
Biologics Technology Manager
Medtronic Sofamor Danek, Inc.
Memphis, Tennessee

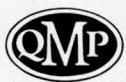

Quality Medical Publishing, Inc.
ST. LOUIS, MISSOURI
2006

Copyright © 2006 by Quality Medical Publishing, Inc.

All rights reserved. No part of this publication may be reproduced, stored in a retrieval system, or transmitted in any form or by any means, electronic, mechanical, photocopying, recording, or otherwise, without prior permission of the publisher.

Printed in Canada

This book presents current scientific information and opinion pertinent to medical professionals. It does not provide advice concerning specific diagnosis and treatment of individual cases. It is not intended for use by the layperson. Medical knowledge is constantly changing. As new information becomes available, changes in treatment, procedures, equipment, and the use of drugs and devices sometimes become necessary. The editors/authors/contributors and the publisher have, as far as it is possible, taken care to ensure that the information given in this text is accurate and up to date. Before use, healthcare professionals should read and follow all product package inserts for the country (e.g., Canada or the United States). Information contained in this book is in whole or in part from the FDA Summary of Safety and Effectiveness Data, published July 2, 2002. However, readers are strongly advised to confirm that the information, especially with regard to drug usage, complies with the latest legislation and standards of practice. The authors and publisher will not be responsible for any errors or liable for actions taken as a result of information or opinions expressed in this book.

Quality Medical Publishing, Inc.
2248 Welsch Industrial Court
St. Louis, Missouri 63146
Telephone: 800-348-7808, 314-878-7808
Website: *http://www.qmp.com*

LIBRARY OF CONGRESS CATALOGING-IN-PUBLICATION DATA

McKay, William F.
    The science of rhBMP-2 / William F. McKay, Steven M. Peckham, James S. Marotta.
        p. ; cm.
Includes bibliographical references and index.
ISBN 1-57626-153-0
1. Bone-grafting. 2. Bone morphogenetic proteins—Therapeutic use—Testing.
I. Peckham, Steven M. II. Manager, Biologics Research and Development.
    [DNLM: 1. Bone Morphogenetic Proteins—standards. 2. Bone Morphogenetic Proteins—therapeutic use. 3. Bone Transplantation—methods. WE 190 M478r 2006]
RD123 .M38 2006
617.4′710592—dc21

PREFACE

Bone morphogenetic protein (BMP) was first isolated from bone almost 20 years ago. Most of the work, including safety, toxicity, and efficacy testing of the individual BMPs after they were isolated, was conducted in the laboratories of industry. With FDA clearance of rhBMP-2 (INFUSE® Bone Graft) as a bone graft replacement through a Pre-Market Approval (PMA) process and the commercial availability of INFUSE® Bone Graft for more than 3 years, it is important to share some of the unpublished data to better educate surgeons, researchers, and patients about this technology.

It would take years to publish all the safety and toxicity studies, and the data would be dispersed throughout the literature. Thus, this book was written to compile this body of work into a single resource to help the reader better understand the scope and breadth of safety, toxicity, and efficacy testing that has been performed with rhBMP-2 and the clean safety profile of this protein. In addition, the interaction of the rhBMP-2 protein with its carrier will be better understood, helping to ensure its proper clinical use.

The Science of rhBMP-2 explains the need for autograft replacement technology, the differences among various bone grafting technologies, and how to compare and contrast these technologies to distinguish the good from the poor (but heavily marketed) technologies. The balance of the book focuses on rhBMP-2 technology, which is the most extensively researched technology in orthopedic history, reflecting its revolutionary contribution to orthopedics.

Autograft replacement technology has already helped thousands of patients to date, and many more will benefit from its use in the future as new rhBMP-2 carriers and indications are developed.

William F. McKay, ME
Steven M. Peckham, PhD
James S. Marotta, PhD

Acknowledgments

We would like to acknowledge Medtronic Sofamor Danek's business partner, Wyeth, for their contribution of much of the safety and toxicity data for this book. In particular, we wish to thank John Wozney, Rod Riedel, and MaryLou Bell at Wyeth, who devoted much of their careers to discovering rhBMP-2 and developing it into the commercial product it is today.

At Medtronic Sofamor Danek, many individuals also devoted significant time turning rhBMP-2 into a product surgeons could use clinically and gaining FDA clearance to ultimately put the product into surgeons' hands. Among these are Rick Treharne, Bailey Lipscomb, Tara Hood, Debbie Desrochers, and Judy English.

Medtronic Sofamor Danek would like to recognize the many surgeons for their significant contributions to the clinical study of rhBMP-2 that led to FDA approval of INFUSE® Bone Graft and helped introduce this revolutionary technology to the world of medicine.

Contents

Chapter 1 *Graft Replacements* 1

The Need for Graft Replacements 2
Spinal Fusion Graft Requirements 2
Challenges of Spinal Fusion Grafts 3
The Rationale for Iliac Crest Bone as the Current Standard of Care 4
Limitations of Local Autograft Bone (Compared With Iliac Crest Bone) 5
Bone Graft Extender/Replacement Options 5
Osteoconductive Versus Osteoinductive Materials 8
The Role and Importance of Osteoinductivity for Spinal Fusion Graft Materials 9
Assays for Osteoinductivity 10
DBM Versus BMP 12
Criteria (Burden of Proof) for Spinal Fusion Graft Replacements 14
Frequently Asked Questions 16

Chapter 2 *BMP Basics* 23

Background on BMP Discovery 24
Definition and Description 26
Types of BMPs and Their Respective Roles 26
Role of BMP in Bone Repair and Formation 27

BMP Versus Other Growth Factors   34
Sources of BMP and Advantages and Limitations
   of Each   35
Frequently Asked Questions   37

Chapter 3   *Overview of rhBMP-2*   41

Background and Description of Recombinant Human
   BMP-2 (rhBMP-2)   42
Safety of rhBMP-2   45
Assessment of Carcinogenicity and Toxicity   56
Role of Carrier   58
Rationale and Criteria for rhBMP-2 Carriers   58
Frequently Asked Questions   62

Chapter 4   *rhBMP-2 and ACS*   67

Selection of ACS as rhBMP-2 Carrier   68
Description of ACS   69
Characterization of rhBMP-2 and ACS Binding   70
Safety of rhBMP-2/ACS   73
Mechanisms and Timing of rhBMP-2/ACS–Induced Bone
   Formation   79
Frequently Asked Questions   80

Chapter 5   *Preclinical Efficacy of rhBMP-2 and ACS*   87

Dosage and Concentration Selection   88
Species-Specific BMP Healing Rates   90
Techniques for Evaluating Spinal Fusions   92

Preclinical rhBMP-2/ACS Interbody Studies With Metal
   Cages and Allograft Bone Dowels   93
Comparisons With Iliac Crest Autograft: Rate and Quality
   of Fusion   100
Limitations of the Compressible Collagen Sponge
   Carrier   101
rhBMP-2 as a Possible Graft Enhancer   106
Preclinical rhBMP-2 Posterolateral Studies: Use of Bulking
   Agents   108
Effect on Spinal Tissue   110
Frequently Asked Questions   114

Chapter 6   *Clinical Efficacy of rhBMP-2/ACS*   117

INFUSE® Bone Graft/LT-CAGE® Lumbar Tapered Fusion
   Device Description   118
INFUSE® Bone Graft/LT-CAGE® Lumbar Tapered Fusion
   Device Pilot Clinical Study Results   121
INFUSE® Bone Graft/LT-CAGE® Lumbar Tapered Fusion
   Device Pivotal Clinical Study Results   128
Frequently Asked Questions   135

Index   139

THE SCIENCE OF rhBMP-2

CHAPTER 1

Graft Replacements

 ## The Need for Graft Replacements

It is estimated that more than 300,000 spinal fusion procedures are performed each year in the United States. The success or failure of these procedures depends on a combination of the mechanical stabilization that spinal hardware provides during the short term and the biologic fusion that a bone graft material provides over the longer term. Biologic fusion is the result of new bone formation at the fusion site. In the absence of a biologic fusion mass, the spinal hardware may eventually fail. Surgeons have always had control over short-term mechanical stabilization, but have lacked the capacity to produce a consistent biologic fusion. The current "gold standard" bone graft material used in spinal fusion is autologous bone harvested from the iliac crest. The morbidity and lack of consistent biologic fusion associated with iliac crest bone grafts have led to research for new bone graft substitutes for use in spinal fusions.

 ## Spinal Fusion Graft Requirements

Some requirements for a bone graft substitute have become evident. The bone graft substitute must be able to produce a good fusion similar or superior to that produced by iliac crest autograft. Healthy autograft provides osteoprogenitor cells and the inductive agents necessary to produce new bone. Autograft quality varies with the health and age of the patient. A bone graft substitute needs to be of consistent quality and capability to produce fusion. It must be biocompatible and safe for human use. In addition, spinal fusions require additional mechanical stability, and advances in spinal instrumentation have increased success rates for lumbar spinal fusion procedures. Bone grafting in the lumbar spine is generally more complicated than in other clinical applications, and consequently, the requirements for graft replacements are more stringent.

Understanding the process by which bone forms, heals, and remodels is a prerequisite to finding the best bone grafting material. New bone formation requires a scaffold for early osteoid (unmineralized) bone deposition, which eventually undergoes ossification. This scaffold acts as the initial bridge between bone surfaces that are attempting to unite. In normal fracture healing, the scaffold consists of a fibrin and collagen matrix, which forms the callus around a fractured bone. Most long bone fractures produce small gaps that are easily healed by the body. However, large gaps or distances may need to be bridged after surgical procedures or more severe fractures. In such cases, a surgically placed scaffold may promote the body's own healing potential.

Challenges of Spinal Fusion Grafts

There are clear problems associated with achieving successful lumbar spinal fusions in humans. Up to 40% of patients have been reported to develop nonunions, or failure to achieve a solid bony fusion.[1] A spinal nonunion usually leaves the clinical symptoms unresolved, providing an unsatisfactory experience for the patient, and frequently resulting in a second surgery. Therefore improving the spinal fusion success rate continues to be a surgical goal. One area that has been the subject of much research, because of its potential for improving fusion rates, is the development of clinically effective bone graft substitutes.

Developing grafting options for lumbar spinal fusions requires good animal models for preclinical studies. The animal models must have fusion rates similar to those reported in humans, while dealing with surgical constraints similar to those expected in clinical applications.

To further validate the efficacy of various bone graft options, advancements in evaluating the fusion mass had to be made. One valuable tool for assessing the quality of fusion is histology of a complete section through the fusion mass; however, histologic sections of this magnitude are not possible in humans. Additionally, studies have shown that even standard radiographic imaging methods may be insufficient for determining if solid fusions have developed.[2,3] Clearly, improved radiographic methods were required to accurately assess the efficacy of autogenous bone graft replacements.

The Rationale for Iliac Crest Bone as the Current Standard of Care

Iliac crest bone is usually an excellent source of autogenous bone graft material. Autograft bone provides growth factors necessary to initiate and facilitate the production of new bone and usually provides enough volume for multiple-level spinal fusion without compromising the strength of the hip. Autograft harvesting requires an additional surgery, which is frequently the cause for both immediate and long-term pain and other problems for the patient. Years of experience with fusion success using iliac crest bone have provided a high standard and taught us what to look for in a replacement.

Limitations of Local Autograft Bone (Compared With Iliac Crest Bone)

Local autograft bone derived from laminae, facet joints, and/or spinous processes is sometimes used as the bone graft source in lumbar spinal fusion. It is also sometimes supplemented with allograft bone if there is not sufficient bone present to provide the needed volume for the graft. However, local spinal bone lacks the rich supply of bone marrow and osteogenic potential available in iliac crest bone. Moreover, local bone supply is usually of inadequate quantity to provide good fusion. In most spinal lumbar fusions, the iliac crest is the preferred graft. To date, there have been no clinical studies comparing the quality of spinal fusion with iliac crest bone versus local autograft bone.

Bone Graft Extender/Replacement Options

Based largely on their osteoinductive potential, bone grafting materials can generally be classified as either bone graft replacements or bone graft extenders. The osteoinductive potential of bone graft extenders ranges from minimal (e.g., allograft products) to none (e.g., ceramics); therefore these are only used to extend or supplement iliac crest bone graft, which provides the necessary osteoinductive factors to initiate new bone formation and fusion. Bone graft extenders added to autograft bone act as osteoconductive scaffolding to bridge gaps between the autograft bone chips. Only a relatively small amount of extender material should be added to autograft (approximately 25%) to ensure fusion success. If autograft chips become separated by gaps that are too large, the autograft's osteoinductivity will be insufficient to reach across the osteoconductive scaffold to connect all the autograft chips. The use of demineralized bone matrix (DBM) as a bone graft extender, a type of allograft, provides the advantage of some minimal osteoinductivity to facilitate this bridging of new bone between the autograft chips. Ceramics do not have any bone-forming capacity and are less likely to facilitate this fusion process.

A number of additional bone graft extender products are either available on the market or undergoing development for use in the spine. These materials range from synthetic ceramics to demineralized bone matrix products and bone marrow or patient blood-derived products. The selection is broad, but they primarily offer slightly different degrees of bone graft extender capability, as none of these products are significantly osteoinductive.

Although biomaterials have been developed to act as scaffolds in larger bone defects, they do not in themselves have the capacity to induce new bone formation. This capacity, known as osteoinductivity, is most commonly determined in a rat subcutaneous implant model (Fig. 1-1). If a material is osteoinductive, it should be able to consistently form a bone nodule within two weeks of implantation into a nonbony site. If bone formation takes longer than two weeks, or if the material has to be placed in an intramuscular location to form the bone nodule, it is considered less inductive.[4] Because most biomaterials fail to induce new bone formation, they are categorized as osteoconductive rather than osteoinductive.

Because rats form bone quickly and easily, it is important to further test a material's osteoinductive "potency," or capability, in a higher-order species. In these models, a more potent osteoinductive material is required to promote bone formation. If a material passes these two levels of tests, it is likely to be osteoinductive in human applications.

Figure 1-1

Comparison of osteoconductive to osteoinductive results in an ectopic bone study. After subcutaneous implantation in a rat for 2 weeks, osteoconductive materials do not form new bone, whereas osteoinductive materials do form new bone.

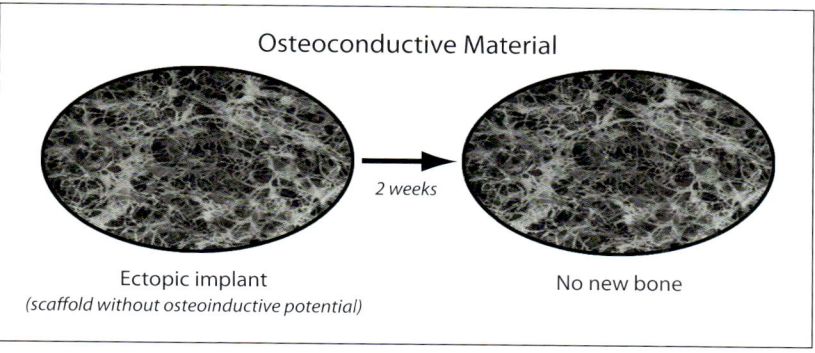

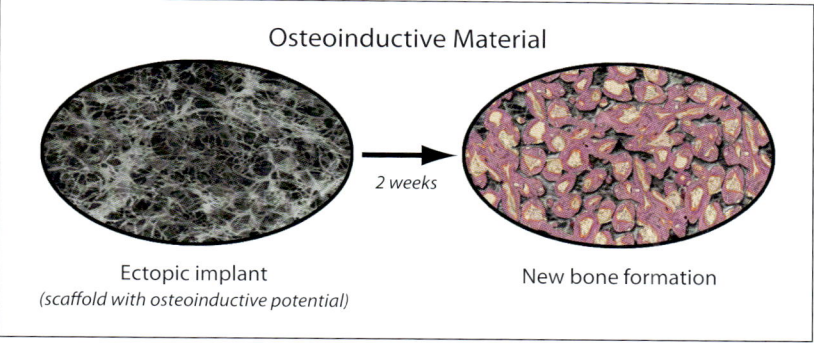

Bone graft replacements possess osteoinductive potential equal to or greater than autogenous bone graft and can therefore be used to eliminate the need for autograft completely. The only known true bone graft replacements are those that contain bone morphogenetic protein (BMP), such as INFUSE® Bone Graft (Medtronic Sofamor Danek, Memphis, TN) which was recently approved by the FDA for use with specific interbody fusion devices (such as the LT-CAGE® and INTER FIX™ devices). INFUSE® Bone Graft consists of recombinant human bone morphogenetic protein-2 (rhBMP-2, known as dibotermin alfa) placed on an absorbable collagen sponge (ACS). The INFUSE® Bone Graft component induces new bone tissue at the site of implantation and is the only clinically proven replacement for autologous iliac crest bone graft.

Bone graft extenders and replacements can be listed in increasing order of osteoinductive potential and likelihood of success:
1. Ceramics
2. Ceramic/collagen composites
3. Bone marrow transplants
4. Allograft DBM
5. Human BMP extracts
6. Recombinant human BMP (rhBMP)

Osteoconductive Versus Osteoinductive Materials

Osteoconductive products are useful only in situations in which adequate components needed for bone formation, such as osteoprogenitor cells, osteoinductive proteins released from bleeding bone surfaces, and a blood supply, are in close proximity to the defect. These products are considered to be bone void fillers (i.e., they are intended to fill defects in bone). They should not be used to treat large defects that, in the surgeon's opinion, would fail to heal spontaneously. If the size of the defect is beyond the body's capacity to supply the necessary components, it is unlikely that an osteoconductive material will be able to promote healing of the bony defect. Therefore osteoconductive materials are only useful in limited applications that are typically less challenging. Their limited application range is expanded when autologous bone graft is added to the osteoconductive material. The percentage of autograft contained in a mixture of autograft/osteoconductive material matrix must be increased in more challenging applications. For example, posterolateral spinal fusions, one of the more complex bone grafting procedures, would probably require a 75%/25% mixture of autograft/osteoconductive matrix.

With the exception of some allograft-derived DBM products, most commercially available bone graft products are considered osteoconductive only. Indeed, cortical allografts are not considered osteoinductive and are only slightly osteoconductive. Allografts, in general, are less osteoinductive and osteoconductive than autografts.[5] Both autografts and allografts exert their osteoinductive nature through the presence of minute amounts of BMP within the graft. The identification and isolation of the family of bone morphogenetic proteins was a clear step forward for promoting bone induction, which will be discussed further in Chapter 2.

The Role and Importance of Osteoinductivity for Spinal Fusion Graft Materials

Although the success rate for autologous iliac crest bone grafts has been reasonable for lumbar spinal fusions, the success rate is by no means 100%. This is the case despite the fact that autograft is clearly osteoinductive in nature. Accepting a less osteoinductive material than autograft as a replacement for autograft would decrease, rather than improve, the success rate of spinal fusion surgery. Lumbar fusions are challenging surgeries even when using fresh autograft. Improving surgical success means improving the osteoinductive capacity of the material, while keeping the osteoconductive ability intact. Bone morphogenetic proteins are the only growth and differentiation factors known to be osteoinductive.

 # Assays for Osteoinductivity

Currently only one validated and accepted method exists for studying the osteoinductivity of materials. Commonly called the *rat ectopic bone assay,* this test was extensively used in the development of osteoinductive materials. Dr. Marshall Urist used this assay when he discovered the existence of bone morphogenetic proteins in bone more than 40 years ago.

Although used in numerous studies, the assay is time consuming and expensive. However, it is an *in vivo* test method that gives clear results indicative of the level of osteoinductivity present in the material undergoing investigation (see Fig. 1-1). The material being tested is implanted subcutaneously and allowed to grow and develop bone. After a few weeks, radiographic images are taken, the material is explanted, and the amount of bone developed is determined by the size of the bone mass. Tests can also be done on the density of bone formed and amount of mineral present. The quality of the bone is usually determined by histology (Fig. 1-2). The only substances identified to date that have been found to be capable of inducing new bone formation at nonbony sites within the time frame of the standard ectopic assay are those that contain bone morphogenetic proteins.

Cell line assays are also being developed to measure osteoinductivity. The most common cell assay involves osteoprogenitor cells. The cell line, called W20, or W20 C17, is a mouse stromal cell line, which is a target cell line for rhBMP-2. The American Society for Testing and Materials (ASTM) has established a method for determining the *in vitro* biologic activity of rhBMP using this cell line.[6] In experiments using this cell line, the cells produce increased alkaline phosphatase activity in response to exposure to rhBMP-2, and its presence is correlated with the ectopic bone-forming capability of rhBMP-2. Alkaline phosphatase is an enzyme associated with the osteogenic activity of bone-forming cells. The assay is performed in the common 96-well microtiter plate format. After exposure to rhBMP-2, the p-nitrophenol generated from the alkaline phosphatase substrate can be measured by optical density in a spectrophotometer. This metric provides a relevant prediction of the bone-forming capacity of rhBMP-2.

There are many obvious reasons, including speed, expense, and reproducibility, which would promote the acceptance of such a method in the scientific community. A cell line assay would be the obvious choice over an implant study when speed is paramount and when incremental differences in activity are being investigated. It would also be more acceptable as a quality-control method during manufacture and purification of rhBMP-2. It should be understood that this ASTM method is an indirect measure of the biologic activity of rhBMP-2, and that it should be regularly validated against an *in vivo* ectopic bone formation model or certified rhBMP-2 standard.

Figure 1-2

The osteoinductive capacity of rhBMP-2/ACS is shown in this rat ectopic model. The subcutaneous implant formed a bone nodule 2 weeks after implantation of rhBMP-2/ACS (not intramuscular). Histologic examination on the right confirms the formation of new bone tissue.

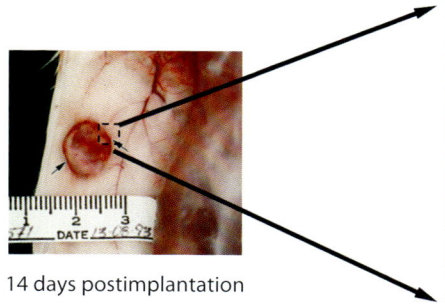

14 days postimplantation

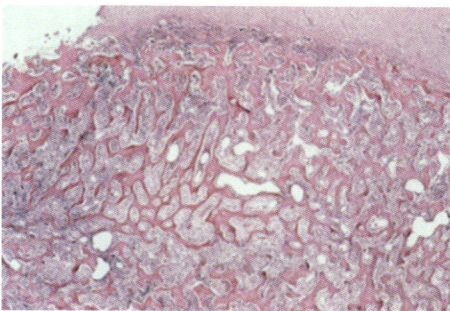

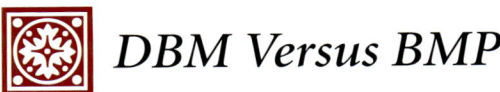 DBM Versus BMP

Demineralized bone matrix (DBM) products will typically form bone in the rat ectopic assay. This is because they contain trace amounts of BMP, and the required threshold level to cause inductivity in the rat model is fairly low. Thus, the rat subcutaneous implant model may not be appropriate to ensure reliable osteoinductivity for human patients. It is uncertain whether the level of BMP in DBM is consistent enough and sufficient to induce consistent bone formation in higher-order animal species or in humans.

Depending on the tissue-processing protocols used by individual tissue banks, different DBM products may contain different levels of BMP and may vary from lot to lot. Blum, et al. recently measured the amount of BMP-2 and TGF-β from 113 different lots of DBM obtained from various tissue banks and found that the BMP-2 concentration ranged between 200 to 6744 pg/g.[7] The authors also found that the area of new bone formed by these DBM products in a rat ectopic assay was directly proportional to the amount of BMP-2 detected (Fig. 1-3). The authors found no association between the amount of TGF-β and the percentage of new bone formed. Quality control testing by most tissue banks is not standardized. From both clinical and research perspectives, the presence of consistent quantities of bone morphogenetic proteins in allograft materials is a significant issue. In the absence of this consistency, the interpretation of both *in vitro* and *in vivo* results will be confounded. The availability of a material with consistent quality and controlled osteoinductivity would be a great advantage to surgeons. Surgeons should know what quality control testing their DBM supplier conducts and demand that every lot of DBM be tested for osteoinductivity.

Figure 1-3

Level of BMP-2 detected in DBM versus the percentage of new bone formation in an athymic nude rat muscle pouch model. Note the linear association between BMP-2 and the amount of new bone formation ($p < 0.0001$). (From Blum B, Moseley J, Miller L, et al. Measurement of bone morphogenetic proteins and other growth factors in demineralized bone matrix. Orthopedics 27[1 Suppl]:S161-S165, 2004.)

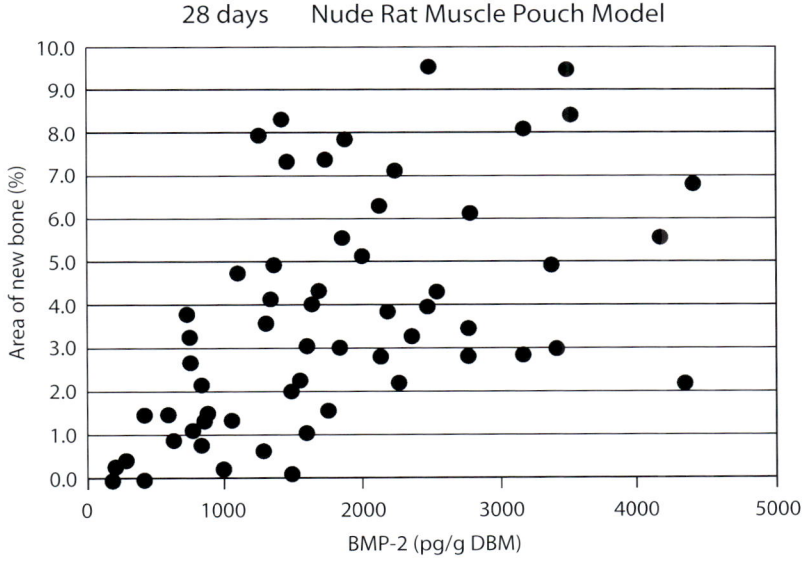

Criteria (Burden of Proof) for Spinal Fusion Graft Replacements

The burden of proof required for clinical efficacy of bone graft replacements is very high. Bone graft substitutes should be expected to meet the minimum-level burden of proof before they are widely used clinically (Fig. 1-4). Minimum requirements for a bone graft substitute are as follows:

1. Induction of ectopic (nonbony site) bone in rats
2. 100% effectiveness in a challenging animal (monkey) spinal fusion model
3. Prospective, randomized clinical data demonstrating safety and effectiveness

Challenging bone graft applications such as lumbar spinal fusions require a sufficient level of osteoinductivity. To ensure that a bone graft is osteoinductive, data must, at a minimum, demonstrate bone formation at an ectopic or nonbony site in rats. Higher osteoinductive potency is indicated by bone formation in a subcutaneous ectopic site as opposed to an intramuscular site and formation within 2 weeks as opposed to a longer time period.

The second burden of proof that a bone graft substitute must satisfy before clinical use is data demonstrating a 100% fusion rate in a higher-order animal model such as a nonhuman primate spinal fusion model. Nonhuman primate models most closely model the slow rate of bone formation in humans and have a high threshold for BMP-induced bone formation. If a bone graft substitute is 100% effective in monkeys, it has a high likelihood of being effective in humans.

Finally, a bone graft substitute must be shown to be safe and effective in a prospective, randomized, controlled clinical trial. The control group should reflect the current standard of care, that is, autologous iliac crest bone graft. Only a prospective, randomized clinical study can scientifically demonstrate the safety and effectiveness of a product.

Figure 1-4

Minimum burden of proof that bone graft substitutes should be expected to meet before they are widely used for spinal fusion. The minimum levels include induction of new bone formation in a rat ectopic model, 100% effectiveness in a challenging animal (nonhuman primate) fusion model, and finally, a prospective, randomized clinical study demonstrating safety and effectiveness.

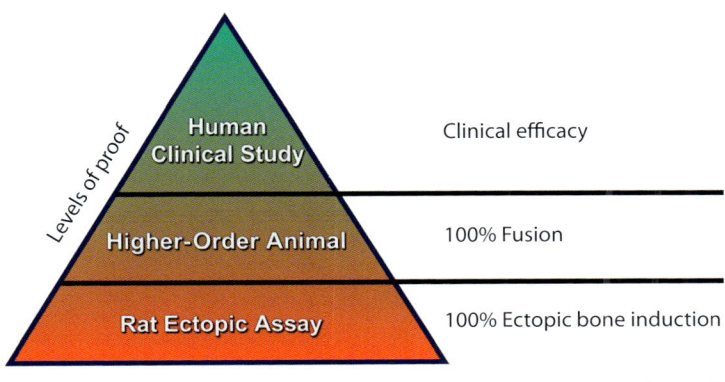

 Frequently Asked Questions

Is the medical community familiar with BMPs?

Both orthopedic surgeons and neurosurgeons have long anticipated the widespread use of BMPs in spinal fusion applications. Dozens of review, preclinical, and clinical papers have been published in orthopedic journals during the last decade, such as the following examples:

> Sandhu HS. Bone morphogenetic proteins and spinal surgery [review]. Spine 28(15 Suppl):S64-S73, 2003.
> McKay B, Sandhu HS. Use of recombinant human bone morphogenetic protein-2 in spinal fusion applications [review]. Spine 27(16 Suppl 1):S66-S85, 2002.

How does the quantity of BMP delivered in INFUSE® Bone Graft compare with autograft bone?

The quantity of BMP available in the autograft bone is much lower. Natural BMP constitutes less than 0.01% of total bone protein and less than 0.001% of the wet weight of marrow-free compact bone. A total dose of 4.2 mg rhBMP-2 would equal 420 g of autograft bone under the very best of circumstances. In addition, a variation in autograft BMP level is associated with health status and age.

What other products contain BMP?

In general, bone graft substitutes can be categorized as either osteoconductive or osteoinductive.

Spinal fusion autograft replacements need to be osteoinductive given the challenge of these procedures. BMPs are the only known osteoinductive differentiation factors.

Demineralized bone matrix (DBM) materials contain BMP but at levels much, much lower than recombinant proteins like INFUSE® Bone Graft. (For example, DBM has approximately 0.000001 mg/ml of BMP, while INFUSE® Bone Graft has 1.5 mg/ml—which is about 1 million times more.) The low concentration of BMP in DBM limits the application of DBM to that of a graft extender.

INFUSE® Bone Graft represents the first osteoinductive spinal fusion graft replacement available for use in the United States.

OP-1® Putty (Stryker Biotech, Hopkinton, MA) is a product that contains recombinant human osteogenic protein-1 (OP-1), also known as recombinant human BMP-7 (rhBMP-7). To date, the clinical results of OP-1® Putty in spinal fusion have not achieved the level of success seen in animal studies and are reporting fusion rates of 65-75% in pilot clinical studies.

How do INFUSE® Bone Graft and OP-1® Putty differ? Does INFUSE® Bone Graft offer specific advantages over OP-1® Putty?

INFUSE® Bone Graft utilizes rhBMP-2, while the OP-1® Putty product uses rhBMP-7. Both proteins have been studied very extensively by the scientific community in general. Both proteins have been shown to be osteoinductive. However, they are fundamentally different proteins, which are placed in different subgroups among the numerous BMPs discovered so far. For example, rhBMP-7 has been shown to be systemically available, while rhBMP-2 is not.

OP-1® Putty has an FDA humanitarian device exemption (HDE), which is not the same as a full pre-market approval (PMA). OP-1® Putty is authorized by federal law for use as an alternative to autograft in compromised patients requiring revision posterolateral (intertransverse) lumbar spinal fusion, for whom harvest of autologous bone or bone marrow is not feasible or is not expected to promote fusion. Examples of compromising factors include osteoporosis, smoking, and diabetes. The effectiveness of OP-1® Putty for this use has not been demonstrated. It is interesting to note that the study used to determine the probable benefit of OP-1® Putty involved primary posterolateral spinal fusion and not revision spinal fusion. This study also excluded smokers and obese patients.

INFUSE® Bone Graft has an FDA approval as a replacement for autograft in anterior lumbar interbody fusion (ALIF) using either the LT-CAGE® Device, INTER FIX™ Cage, or INTER FIX™ RP Cage. The

Table 1-1

Comparison of INFUSE® Bone Graft and OP-1® Putty

	INFUSE® Bone Graft	OP-1® Putty
Protein	rhBMP-2	rhBMP-7
BMP delivered	Four kits: 4.2 to 12 mg	3.5 mg
Carrier	2.8 to 8.0 cc collagen sponge	1 g collagen granules and 230 mg carboxymethyl cellulose (CMC)
BMP concentration	1.5 mg/ml	0.88 mg/ml
Indication	ALIF with LT-CAGE® or INTERFIX™ fusion device	Compromised patients requiring revision posterolateral lumbar fusion
Regulatory status	PMA Proven clinically effective	HDE Efficacy not proven
Price	$3600 to $5000	$11,000 for 2 kits
Clinical success	94.5% Fusion success 55% Improvement in Oswestry score	63% Bilateral fusion success NOTE: Study investigated the use of OP-1® Putty in primary posterolateral spine fusions (not revisions)

INFUSE® Bone Graft is available in four different kit sizes designed to match with the various cages for which it is approved. OP-1® Putty is available in one kit size and its HDE indication requires that two kits be used for a bilateral spine fusion.

ALIF, Anterior lumbar interbody fusion; *HDE*, humanitarian device exemption; *PMA*, pre-market approval.

safety and efficacy of INFUSE® Bone Graft for this indication has been demonstrated in order to gain FDA approval. Additional differences between the two products are listed in Table 1-1.

How does the approval of a BMP product affect the use of demineralized bone matrix?

Demineralized bone matrix is a source of BMP that is derived from pulverized bone specimens and is typically used as a bone grafting material. The amount of BMP in DBM varies widely from lot to lot (see Fig. 1-3). Processing may also destroy or inactivate the BMP found in DBM. Since DBM contains low concentrations of BMP, it has often produced disappointing results in clinical studies. The approval of rhBMP-2 provides a positive alternative for patients initially diagnosed as candidates for fusion using demineralized bone matrix, since it is a pure BMP-2 protein. DBM may still be mixed with autologous iliac crest bone to extend the volume of the final graft or used in less challenging fusion environments such as a single-level anterior cervical fusion. DBM is not indicated as an autograft replacement.

What is an HDE?

According to the Food and Drug Administration's guide, "Humanitarian Device Exemptions (HDE) Regulation: Questions and Answers; Final Guidance for Industry"[8]:

> A Humanitarian Device Exemption (HDE) is an application that is similar to a PMA application but is exempt from the effectiveness requirements of a PMA. An approved HDE authorizes marketing of a Humanitarian Use Device (HUD). As defined in the Federal Food, Drug, and Cosmetic Act, a HUD is a device that is "intended to benefit patients in the treatment and diagnosis of diseases or conditions that affect fewer than 4,000 individuals in the United States." In the final regulation, however, the FDA added the qualifying phrase "per year" to the defining criteria. As the agency explained in the preamble to the final rule, the FDA believes that "a point prevalence definition would be considerably more restrictive and provide less of an incentive for the development of such devices." The FDA also added the phrase "or is

manifested" to the definition of a HUD "to establish that [a] HUD designation may be appropriate in cases where more than 4,000 people have the disease but fewer than 4,000 manifest the condition" (61 FR 33233, June 26, 1996). Therefore the final definition of a HUD is a device that is intended to benefit patients in the treatment and diagnosis of diseases or conditions that affect or [are] manifested in fewer than 4,000 individuals in the United States per year.

Can a product with HDE approval be used off-label?

According to the FDA guide[8]:

> Because Institutional Review Board (IRB) review and approval is required before an HDE product is used within its approved labeling, it should not be used outside of its approved labeling without similar restrictions. That is, in an emergency situation, a HUD may be used off-label to save the life or protect the physical well-being of a patient, but the physician . . . should follow the emergency use procedures governing such use of unapproved devices. . . . Before the device is used, if possible, the physician should obtain the IRB chairperson's concurrence, informed consent from the patient . . . and an independent assessment by an uninvolved physician.

Why is IRB approval required before using a product with HDE approval?

IRB review and approval of a HUD is required by the FDA. The healthcare provider is responsible for obtaining IRB approval before the product is implanted in a patient. IRBs are responsible for initial as well as continuing review of the HDE product. IRBs should be cognizant that the use of the device should not exceed the scope of the FDA-approved indication.

REFERENCES

1. Steinmann JC, Herkowitz HN. Pseudarthrosis of the spine [review]. Clin Orthop Relat Res 284:80-90, 1992.
2. Brodsky AE, Kovalsky ES, Khalil MA. Correlation of radiologic assessment of lumbar spine fusions with surgical exploration. Spine 16(6 Suppl):S261-S265, 1991.
3. Dawson EG, Clader TJ, Bassett LW. A comparison of different methods used to diagnose pseudarthrosis following posterior spinal fusion for scoliosis. J Bone Joint Surg Am 67:1153-1159, 1985.

4. Yoshida K, Bessho K, Fujimura K, et al. Osteoinduction capability of recombinant human bone morphogenetic protein-2 in intramuscular and subcutaneous sites: An experimental study. J Craniomaxillofac Surg 26:112-115, 1998.
5. Greenwald AS, Boden SD, Goldberg VM, Khan Y, Laurencin CT, Rosier RN; American Academy of Orthopaedic Surgeons. The Committee on Biological Implants. Bone-graft substitutes: Facts, fictions, and applications. J Bone Joint Surg Am 83(Suppl 2 Pt 2):98-103, 2001.
6. ASTM International. F2131-02 Standard Test Method for in vitro biological activity of recombinant human bone morphogenetic protein-2 (rhBMP-2) using the W-20 mouse stromal cell line. Book of Standards Volume 13.01.
7. Blum B, Moseley J, Miller L, et al. Measurement of bone morphogenetic proteins and other growth factors in demineralized bone matrix. Orthopedics 27(1 Suppl):S161-S165, 2004.
8. Humanitarian Device Exemptions (HDE) Regulation: Questions and answers; final guidance for industry. Food and Drug Administration web site. Document issued on July 12, 2001. Available at *http://www.fda.gov/cdrh/ode/guidance/1381.html*.

CHAPTER 2

BMP Basics

Background on BMP Discovery

Bone healing is an ancient medical art. While small gaps in bone can heal easily on their own, large gaps present considerable healing challenges. The search for an ideal material for bone grafting applications began more than 100 years ago. As early as 1901, there were reports of the use of autologous cancellous bone from the finger for grafting a cleft maxilla.[1] Albee[2] and Hibbs[3] independently published their experiences using autologous bone in the spine in 1911. Iliac crest autograft eventually became the "gold standard" for bone grafting procedures despite widespread recognition of the morbidity associated with bone harvesting.[4-8]

The merits of autologous bone transplantation became clear long before the mechanism by which an autologous graft stimulated new bone growth was understood. The merits include availability, lack of immunogenicity, and excellent bone regrowth when compared with other graft materials. Autologous bone is, therefore, an almost ideal bone grafting material.

As sufficient amounts of quality autologous bone may not be available for grafting, or the autologous bone may be diseased, the need for other materials for bone grafting becomes obvious. Medical researchers have investigated a number of different technologies, most commonly allografts that have some osteoinductive factors that stimulate normal bone growth. However, allografts are not as effective as autografts.[9] The search for a material equal or superior to autologous bone has been an ongoing research goal.

The discovery in 1965 of the family of bone morphogenetic proteins (BMPs), represents the seminal event in the search for an ideal bone graft replacement. Dr. Marshall Urist[10] implanted demineralized bone matrix into the muscle of rabbits, rats, mice, and guinea pigs and found that it induced new bone formation. Bone is about 65% to 70% mineral and 30% to 35% organic matrix. By using a demineralized material, Urist was, in effect, implanting only the organic bone matrix. This organic matrix consists primarily of collagen combined with a number of carbohydrates and other proteins (Fig. 2-1). Further investigation of the noncollagenous proteins found in the bone matrix revealed that a series of proteins, collectively known as bone morphogenetic proteins, were responsible for the *de novo* bone formation observed by Urist.[10-15]

Figure 2-1

Bone consists of both mineral and organic components. Demineralization of bone yields an organic matrix containing collagen and other proteins. The osteoinductive potential of demineralized bone was found to be related to naturally occurring noncollagenous glycoproteins. These osteoinductive glycoproteins are called bone morphogenetic proteins (BMPs).

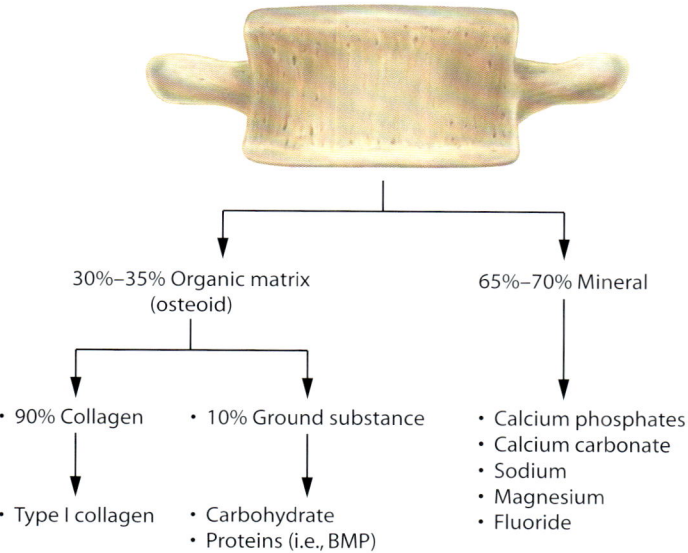

 ## Definition and Description

The interest in bone formation and the ongoing search for a substitute for iliac crest autograft that could induce bone formation without the morbidity associated with graft harvest led to the discovery of BMPs. BMPs are the only proteins known to have the osteoinductive capacity to induce new bone formation. They have been shown to play a role in inducing bone formation during skeletal development[16] and fracture repair.[17] In addition, the osteoinductive properties of autologous bone graft or demineralized bone matrix (DBM) are caused by the action of naturally occurring BMPs.

BMPs belong to the transforming growth factor-β (TGF-β) superfamily of proteins and are related to each other by similarities in amino acid structure. Through the analysis of bone extracts, BMP-2 was identified as one of the osteoinductive factors present in bone.[14] Like other members of the TGF-β superfamily, BMP-2 originates inside the cell in precursor form. The precursor protein undergoes processing within the cell and is secreted as a mature protein. BMP-2 is a locally acting growth and differentiation factor.

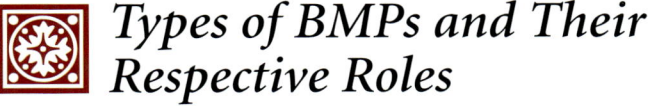 ## Types of BMPs and Their Respective Roles

The primary amino acid structure of BMP-2 is highly conserved across a range of species, suggesting an important role in biologic processes. Although all BMPs are members of the TGF-β superfamily, the proteins are not identical in structure or function and should not be viewed as interchangeable. Significant similarities in amino acid sequence do exist among all BMPs in the carboxy-terminal region of the proteins, and the degree of similarity (or homology) allows the proteins to be grouped into sets. For example, the amino acid structure of BMP-2 is most similar to BMP-4. BMP-5, BMP-6, and BMP-7 share significant homology and are generally considered to be a separate group from the other BMPs.[16] Despite the fact that the abilities of the osteoinductive BMPs to induce bone appear to be qualitatively similar, the *in vivo* developmental and repair mechanisms of the individual BMPs are likely not identical. *In vitro* testing has shown that cells do not all respond in the same way to different BMPs. For example, in one study, BMP-2 stimulated migration of human osteoblasts, whereas BMP-4 and BMP-6 had no effect on cellular migration.[18] In another set of studies, BMP-7 was shown to induce proliferation of the human osteosarcoma cell line TE85, whereas BMP-2 appears to have no effect on these cells.[19] Direct comparison of different BMPs is complicated by the fact that the range of BMPs has rarely been investigated in the same experiments by the same investigators.

Role of BMP in Bone Repair and Formation

The osteoinductive activity of BMPs has exciting implications in spinal fusion procedures. It is this function as a bone grafting material that will be emphasized here. BMPs initiate a complex, multistage cascade of events in promoting *in vivo* bone formation and exert a number of effects on different cell types. BMPs have been shown in both *in vivo* and *in vitro* studies to induce chemotaxis (stimulation of cell migration in response to a chemical signal), cell proliferation, and cell differentiation.[19] As previously mentioned, a significant amount of the research on BMPs has been performed to elucidate the effects of individual BMPs at the cellular level.

The series of events resulting in bone formation in the ectopic rat model has been studied through histologic analysis at various time points after implantation of a demineralized bone matrix.[20] The first three days following implantation are characterized by infiltration and proliferation of mesenchymal cells (Fig. 2-2). Mesenchymal stem cells are undifferentiated, multipotent cells found in bone marrow and, to a lesser degree, in muscle and soft tissue. When properly stimulated, mesenchymal stem cells are capable of becoming any of a number of different cell types. During days four through seven, the stem cells differentiate into chondroblasts and chondrocytes, and cartilage is formed at the implant site. By day 10, the cartilage has matured and calcified. Over the next couple of days, bone cells appear within the implant and begin laying down bone matrix. Mineralization of the bone occurs, and concurrent with the new bone formation, the cartilage template is resorbed. The bone continues to remodel so that eventually only an ossicle of bone remains.

BMP-2 has been shown to be capable of inducing cell migration, proliferation, and differentiation *in vitro*; therefore, BMP-2 may be involved in every stage of *in vivo* bone formation. During the first steps in bone formation, mesenchymal stem cells (MSC), osteoprogenitor cells, and osteoblasts respond to the chemical signals that are normally released in response to bone injury and migrate to the area of osteogenesis (Fig. 2-3). This stimulation of cell migration in response to a chemical signal is known as chemotaxis. BMP-2 can stimulate this migration of cells since it has been shown *in vitro* to be chemotactic for stromal osteoblasts and mature osteoblasts.[18,19] Human osteoblast migration has been shown to be stimulated in a dose-dependent manner by BMP-2. Moreover, investigations have shown that the migration of human MSCs is also directly stimulated by BMP-2. The chemotactic response of these cells was shown to significantly increase with BMP-2 concentration ($p = 0.05$).[18] Only

Figure 2-2

Time line for endochondral bone formation in the rat ectopic assay. Bone formation occurs within 2 weeks after implantation of a matrix containing osteoinductive BMP.

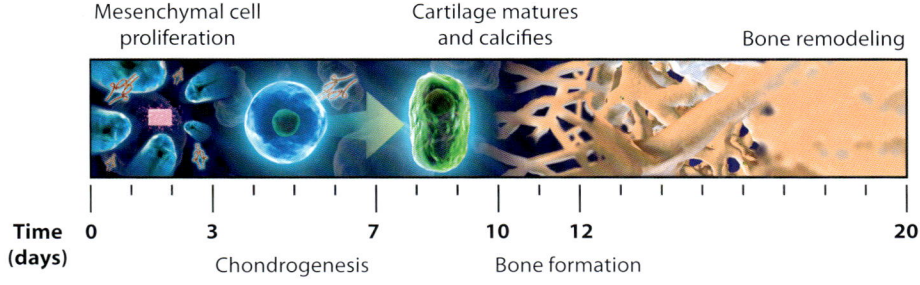

Figure 2-3

Chemotaxis is migration of a cell in response to a chemical signal. Generally, this migration is in the direction of the chemical gradient, that is, from an area of lower concentration to an area of higher concentration. BMP-2 has been shown to be chemotactic for stromal cells and mature osteoblasts in vitro. As BMP is released from a matrix, a concentration gradient can be established that leads to migration of cells to the implant area.

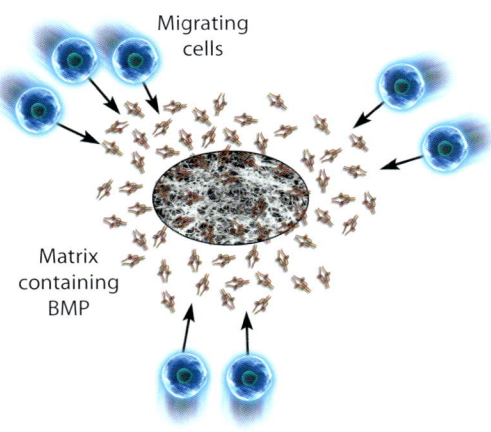

viable cells are capable of chemotactic migration. The viability of cells in transplanted bone marrow aspirate cannot be ensured; therefore, the chemotactic effect of bone marrow aspirate remains questionable. Without this effect, the presence of bone-forming cells at the implant site would be limited.

As the cells migrate into the area, they begin to proliferate (Fig. 2-4). This proliferation can be enhanced by mitogenic factors present at the site of injury or at the graft site. BMP-2 has been shown to have no effect on proliferation of many different committed cell types, including that of an osteosarcoma cell line.[21] On the other hand, BMP-2 has been shown to cause the proliferation of undifferentiated cells. In an *in vitro* cell culture study, BMP-2 increased the proliferation of a multipotent cell line (C26) that is capable of differentiating into osteoblasts, myoblasts, or adipocytes.[22] In that study, BMP-2 also induced differentiation of the C26 cells into osteoblasts, and it inhibited proliferation of a more differentiated osteoblast cell line. Therefore BMP-2 may have a cell-specific effect on the proliferation of multipotent undifferentiated stem cells, but not on mature differentiated cells.

 Figure 2-4

BMPs may act as mitogenic factors. Mitogenic factors stimulate cell division and proliferation. In vitro studies have shown that exposure to BMP-2 results in the cell-specific proliferation of undifferentiated mesenchymal stem cells.

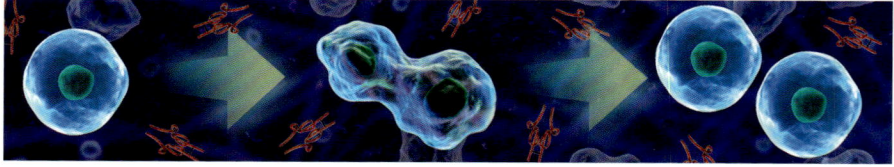

One stem cell divides into two stem cells

The most important function of BMPs in bone formation and the one that is unique to this group of morphogenetic proteins is the induction of cell differentiation. With proper stimuli, mesenchymal stem cells can differentiate into a number of different cell types, including osteoblasts, chondroblasts, and fibroblasts (Fig. 2-5). BMPs direct cell differentiation

Figure 2-5

Mesenchymal stem cells are undifferentiated cells capable of becoming one of a number of connective tissue cells. Of greatest importance with regard to bone formation is the ability of these cells to become bone-producing osteoblasts and cartilage-producing chondrocytes.

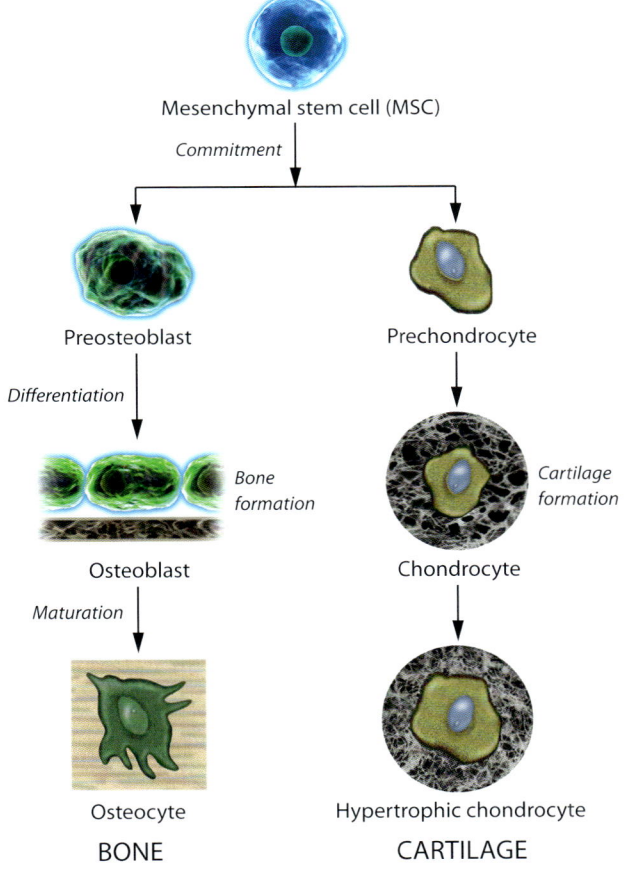

Figure 2-6

Mesenchymal stem cells have specific receptors that recognize and bind to BMPs. Binding of BMP to these receptors initiates an intracellular signaling pathway that leads to differentiation of the stem cell into a bone-producing osteoblast.

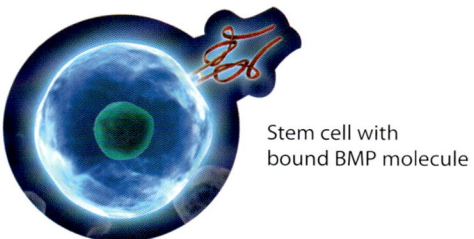

Stem cell with bound BMP molecule

---

by binding to receptors on these cells (Fig. 2-6). Two types of BMP receptors (types I and II) have been identified, and both are able to bind BMPs individually.[23] Most frequently, a heteromeric complex composed of a dimeric BMP bound to BMPRI and BMPRIIB induces cell differentiation. Depending on the BMP, the cell type, and the total environment, chondroblasts or osteoblasts may be formed. This ability to stimulate differentiation of cells is the hallmark of the osteoinductive BMPs. A number of studies have demonstrated the ability of BMP-2 to stimulate the differentiation of multipotent cells into osteoblasts or chondrocytes, depending on the cell type or *in vitro* culture conditions.[22,24,25]

Recently a cell culture study was conducted to compare the osteogenic activity of fourteen recombinant human BMPs directly within a single experiment.[26] Three cell lines, each representing one of the distinct stages of osteoblast differentiation, were tested. Alkaline phosphatase activity was significantly increased in all three cell lines by BMP-2, 6 and 9. The authors concluded that BMP-2, 6, and 9 may be the most potent agents

Figure 2-7

Comprehensive analysis of the osteogenic activity of 14 different BMPs has shown that BMP-2, -6, and -9 play an important role in inducing osteoblast differentiation of mesenchymal stem cells.

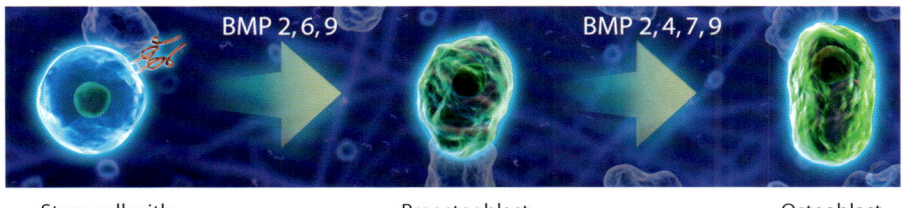

Stem cell with bound BMP molecule — Preosteoblast — Osteoblast

for inducing osteoblast lineage-specific differentiation of mesenchymal stem cells (Fig. 2-7). The observation that BMP-7 exhibited little osteogenic activity in osteoprogenitor cell lines was found by the authors to be "consistent with the relatively moderate success of rhBMP-7 (i.e., OP-1® [Stryker Biotech, Allendale, NJ]) in a recent clinical trial."

During bone formation, BMP-2 plays a vital role in a complicated cascade of events that involves a number of different stimulatory factors and cell types. When BMP-2 is implanted in an ectopic rat model or used as a graft material in a clinical application, the protein does not act independently of all other factors. Although BMP-2 exhibits direct action in recruiting cells to the area and stimulating cell differentiation, the natural biology of bone formation remains intact. The newly recruited and differentiated osteoblasts release proteins, including additional BMP-2 and other factors, to continue to stimulate bone growth and remodeling long after the original implantation of BMP-2. BMP-2 is therefore thought to initiate, stimulate, and amplify the normal bone formation cascade.

BMP Versus Other Growth Factors

Autologous blood-derived products that have recently become commercially available do not contain BMP and have not been shown to be capable of inducing bone growth in the standard rat subcutaneous implant model of osteoinductivity.

The rat develops bone quickly and extensively in response to very low levels of bone morphogenetic proteins; therefore, the presence of any osteoinductive BMPs in the bone graft substitute should be clearly demonstrated in the assay. A study conducted using the rat ectopic assay demonstrated that platelet-rich plasma was not osteoinductive, nor was it able to improve the activity of DBM or DBM with mineralized bone powder.[27] TGF-β factors are present in plasma in concentrations of 100 ng/g, are available from DBM in concentrations of 10,000 ng/g, and probably are not present in sufficient concentration in platelets to facilitate bone formation.[28]

A recent cell culture study was conducted comparing the osteogenic differentiation of rat bone marrow cells exposed to either platelet-rich plasma (PRP) or recombinant human BMP-2.[29] PRP-exposed cultures showed a dose-dependent reduction in alkaline phosphatase activity and calcium deposition, while rhBMP-2 led to the opposite cellular response. The authors concluded that PRP inhibited the osteogenic differentiation of marrow cells and is not a substitute for rhBMP-2 for induction of new bone formation. These findings are further supported by the results of three separate clinical studies which compared spinal fusion techniques using either autologous iliac crest bone graft (ICBG) or ICBG mixed with a platelet-rich gel (ICBG + PRP). Weiner and Walker found that addition of the platelet-rich gel led to a significantly lower rate of solid fusion during single-level intertransverse lumbar fusion.[30] The fusion rate for the ICBG group was 24 of 27, or 91%; whereas the fusion rate for the ICBG + PRP group was 18 of 32, or 62%. The authors concluded that they could not recommend the use of concentrated platelet gels for spinal fusion. These results coincide with a similar trend of lower fusion rates when PRP was added to ICBG in two other clinical studies of spinal fusion.[31,32] Both of these research groups concluded that their data did not support the use of platelet gels to supplement autologous bone graft in spinal fusion procedures.

Sources of BMP and Advantages and Limitations of Each

Naturally occurring BMPs can be isolated or extracted from bone and still remain active.[11-13] Bone can be demineralized by chemical treatment, leaving the bone matrix containing collagen and other components. Extracts from this matrix can be selectively purified to give protein mixtures that have osteoinductive activity. Johnson and colleagues first implanted extracts of human BMP mixed with autograft to successfully treat segmental defects in 1988.[33] This study was followed with the use of human BMP extracts and allograft bone to treat femoral nonunions.[34] This was followed in 1989 by a preclinical study involving allograft bone enhanced with human BMP extracts to produce a spinal fusion in dogs.[35] In this bilateral comparison in 13 animals, the BMP level exhibited an increased number and volume of woven bone formations at all time intervals compared with the control level. This preliminary observation concluded that BMP would serve as a useful adjunct in spinal fusions.

The BMP present in human bone is responsible for the mild osteoinductive property of DBM products. However, BMP found in bone is only available in trace amounts.[14] To provide milligram quantities of isolated human BMP, hundreds of kilograms of bone would be required. Consequently, allograft supply limitations would prevent isolation and purification of a BMP from human bone as a viable option for routine medical use.

An alternate source of BMP is animal bone (xenograft). BMPs are highly conserved across different species, so the BMP isolated from animal bone could be used in human applications. This option also has limitations. As with human bone, hundreds of kilograms of bone would be needed to isolate milligram quantities of BMP. The possibility of immunogenicity associated with a less than 100% purified animal protein product would also be a potential concern. Isolation of BMPs from bone extracts, whether from allograft or xenograft tissue, would need to be rigorously controlled and tested to ensure uniformity of the BMP components and consistency of the osteoinductive activity. In addition, there exists the potential for disease transmission from these animal extracts to humans.

The preferred method for obtaining BMP is to manufacture a recombinant version of a naturally occurring BMP using well-established molecular biology techniques. This production method results in extremely pure solutions of a single BMP. Unlike extraction methods, which derive BMP from allograft or xenograft sources, there are no limitations on the amount of protein that can be produced using recombinant techniques. Additionally, recombinant production offers the advantage of tightly controlled manufacturing processes to ensure the consistency, purity, and biologic activity of the final product.

Advantages of Recombinant Production of BMP-2

- Single protein
- Unlimited supply
- Very pure product
- Consistent, controlled process
- Consistent biologic activity

 # Frequently Asked Questions

What is the level of research activity regarding rhBMP-2?

Thousands of research articles have been published regarding various BMPs in general, and a smaller set of articles on rhBMP-2 specifically. It is estimated that at least 150 research articles are published each year on various BMPs.

To date, there have been several clinical studies conducted on rhBMP-2. INFUSE® Bone Graft has more level 1 clinical evidence than any other bone graft.

Are any animal components used in the growth medium for the rhBMP-2 production cells or in the formulation?

No animal components are used to grow the mammalian cells and none of the formulation stabilizers are animal-derived.

How was the rhBMP-2 protein characterized?

A number of different protein methodologies were used to characterize the rhBMP-2 protein. Techniques included size-exclusion chromatography, peptide mapping, SDS-PAGE, and RP-HPLC.

How is rhBMP-2 activated in the cell?

The dimeric protein attaches to the cell membrane, where two specific types of receptors are present. When the receptor/BMP complex forms, a cascade of events starts with phosphorylation/activation of agents that turn on the genes necessary to differentiate mesenchymal cells into bone-forming cells. From that point on, the rhBMP-2 is no longer involved.

REFERENCES

1. Canady JW, Zeitler DP, Thompson SA, et al. Suitability of the iliac crest as a site for harvest of autogenous bone grafts. Cleft Palate Craniofac J 30:579-581, 1993.
2. Albee FM. The classic. Transplantation of a portion of the tibia into the spine for Pott's disease. A preliminary report. JAMA 57: 885, 1911. Clin Orthop Relat Res 87: 5-8, 1972.
3. Hibbs RA. The classic: The original paper appeared in the New York Medical Journal 93:1013, 1911. I. An operation for progressive spinal deformities: A preliminary report of three cases from the service of the orthopaedic hospital. Clin Orthop Relat Res 35:4-8, 1964.
4. Banwart JC, Asher MA, Hassanein RS. Iliac crest bone graft harvest donor site morbidity. A statistical evaluation. Spine 20:1055-1060, 1995.
5. Fernyhough JC, Schimandle JJ, Weigel MC, et al. Chronic donor site pain complicating bone graft harvesting from the posterior iliac crest for spinal fusion. Spine 17: 1474-1480, 1992.
6. Kurz LT, Garfin SR, Booth RE Jr. Harvesting autogenous iliac bone grafts. A review of complications and techniques. Spine 14:1324-1331, 1989.
7. Laurie SW, Kaban LB, Mulliken JB, et al. Donor-site morbidity after harvesting rib and iliac bone. Plast Reconstr Surg 73:933-938, 1984.
8. Summers BN, Eisenstein SM. Donor site pain from the ilium. A complication of lumbar spine fusion. J Bone Joint Surg Br 71:677-680, 1989.

9. Goldberg VM, Stevenson S. Natural history of autografts and allografts. Clin Orthop Relat Res 225:7-16, 1987.
10. Urist MR. Bone: Formation by autoinduction. Science 150:893-899, 1965.
11. Urist MR, Mikulski A, Lietze A. Solubilized and insolubilized bone morphogenetic protein. Proc Natl Acad Sci USA 76:1828-1832, 1979.
12. Celeste AJ, Iannazzi JA, Taylor RC, et al. Identification of transforming growth factor beta family members present in bone-inductive protein purified from bovine bone. Proc Natl Acad Sci USA 87:9843-9847, 1990.
13. Wozney JM, Rosen V, Celeste AJ, et al. Novel regulators of bone formation: Molecular clones and activities. Science 242:1528-1534, 1988.
14. Wang EA, Rosen V, Cordes P, et al. Purification and characterization of other distinct bone-inducing factors. Proc Natl Acad Sci USA 85:9484-9488, 1988.
15. Sampath TK, Coughlin JE, Whetstone RM, et al. Bovine osteogenic protein is composed of dimers of OP-1 and BMP-2A, two members of the transforming growth factor-beta superfamily. J Biol Chem 265:13198-13205, 1990.
16. Wozney JM, Rosen V. Bone morphogenetic protein and bone morphogenetic protein gene family in bone formation and repair [review]. Clin Orthop Relat Res 346:26-37, 1998.
17. Schmitt JM, Hwang K, Winn SR, et al. Bone morphogenetic proteins: An update on basic biology and clinical relevance [review]. J Orthop Res 17:269-278, 1999.
18. Lind M, Eriksen EF, Bunger C. Bone morphogenetic protein-2 but not bone morphogenetic protein-4 and -6 stimulates chemotactic migration of human osteoblasts, human marrow osteoblasts, and U2-OS cells. Bone 18:53-57, 1996.
19. Wozney JM. Bone morphogenetic proteins and their gene expression. In Noda M, ed. Molecular and Cellular Biology of Bone. San Diego: Academic Press, 1993, pp 131-167.
20. Reddi AH. Cell biology and biochemistry of endochondral bone development. Coll Relat Res 1:209-226, 1981.
21. Wozney JM. The bone morphogenetic protein family and osteogenesis [review]. Mol Reprod Dev 32:160-167, 1992.
22. Yamaguchi A, Katagiri T, Ikeda T, et al. Recombinant human bone morphogenetic protein-2 stimulates osteoblastic maturation and inhibits myogenic differentiation in vitro. J Cell Biol 113:681-687, 1991.
23. Attisano L, Carcamo J, Ventura F, et al. Identification of human activin and TGF beta type I receptors that form heteromeric kinase complexes with type II receptors. Cell 75:671-680, 1993.
24. Hiraki Y, Inoue H, Shigeno C, et al. Bone morphogenetic proteins (BMP-2 and BMP-3) promote growth and expression of the differentiated phenotype of rabbit chondrocytes and osteoblastic MC3T3-E1 cells in vitro. J Bone Miner Res 6:1373-1385, 1991.
25. Wang EA. Bone morphogenetic proteins (BMPs): Therapeutic potential in healing bony defects [review]. Trends Biotechnol 11:379-383, 1993.

26. Cheng H, Jiang W, Phillips FM, et al. Osteogenic activity of the fourteen types of human bone morphogenetic proteins (BMPs). J Bone Joint Surg Am 85:1544-1552, 2003. Erratum in J Bone Joint Surg Am 86:141, 2004.
27. Wironen JF, Jaw RY, Fox WC. Platelet-rich plasma is not osteoinductive in a nude rat assay. Presented at the International Conference of Bone Substitutes Davos, Switzerland, Oct 2000.
28. Jaw RY. Presented at the Twenty-fifth Annual Meeting of the American Association of Tissue Banks, 2001.
29. Arpornmaeklong P, Kochel M, Depprich R, et al. Influence of platelet-rich plasma (PRP) on osteogenic differentiation of rat bone marrow stromal cells. An in vitro study. Int J Oral Maxillofac Surg 33:60-70, 2004.
30. Weiner BK, Walker M. Efficacy of autologous growth factors in lumbar intertransverse fusions. Spine 8:1968-1970; discussion 1971, 2003.
31. Anekstein Y, Glassman S, Puno R, Carreon L. Platelet gel (AGF) fails to increase fusion rate. Presented at the Eighteenth Annual Meeting of the North American Spine Society, San Diego, Oct 2003.
32. Castro FP Jr. Role of activated growth factors in lumbar spinal fusions. J Spinal Disord Tech 17:380-384, 2004.
33. Johnson EE, Urist MR, Finerman GA. Repair of segmental defects of the tibia with cancellous bone grafts augmented with human bone morphogenetic protein. A preliminary report. Clin Orthop Relat Res 236:249-257, 1988.
34. Johnson EE, Urist MR. Human bone morphogenetic protein allografting for reconstruction of femoral nonunion. Clin Orthop Relat Res 371:61-74, 2000.
35. Lovell TP, Dawson EG, Nilsson OS, Urist MR. Augmentation of spinal fusion with bone morphogenetic protein in dogs. Clin Orthop Relat Res 243:266-274, 1989.

CHAPTER 3

Overview of rhBMP-2

Background and Description of Recombinant Human BMP-2 (rhBMP-2)

The discovery of natural osteoinductive factors in bone extracts was only the start of a long journey of research. Identification of the individual proteins responsible for the osteoinductive nature of bone extracts was a painstaking task that spanned the period from 1965 to 1988.[1,2] By using a series of extraction and purification steps, scientists were able to identify individual proteins that induce *in vivo* bone formation. This process was complicated by the fact that a time-consuming *in vivo* rat ectopic assay was necessary at each purification step to identify which fractions contained the components responsible for the osteoinductive activity. One of these osteoinductive proteins eventually identified was designated as BMP-2. Once the BMP-2 protein was identified and subsequently characterized, the next step was to identify the gene that encodes the human BMP-2 protein, making the production of a recombinant version of that protein possible.

Following its identification and isolation, the human BMP-2 gene was inserted into the chromosome of a special type of mammalian production cell (Fig. 3-1). This process, called *recombination,* results in the production of recombinant human BMP-2 (rhBMP-2). The production cells are allowed to grow and multiply. The BMP-2 gene that was spliced into the production cell DNA is copied each time the production cell divides. Each new production cell is able to produce rhBMP-2. This process leads to the formation and expansion of a homogeneous production cell population, which is divided into a number of individual samples known as the "cell bank." The cell bank is stored frozen at $-135°$ C until production of rhBMP-2 is needed. This ensures that any problems (such as growth rate consistency) with one sample can be remedied by using another sample stored in the cell bank. These cells will subsequently produce rhBMP-2, because the information provided in the BMP-2 gene is transcribed into m-RNA. The resulting m-RNA is translated into the rhBMP-2 protein by the genetic and metabolic machinery of the mammalian production cell.

Figure 3-1

Production of recombinant human BMP-2 (rhBMP-2). The gene for the BMP-2 protein is placed in a vector and integrated into the DNA of a commonly used mammalian cell line. The mammalian cells containing the BMP-2 gene begin to produce and secrete rhBMP-2 over time. Periodically, samples of the culture medium are removed from the bioreactor and the solution is purified to yield the rhBMP-2 product.

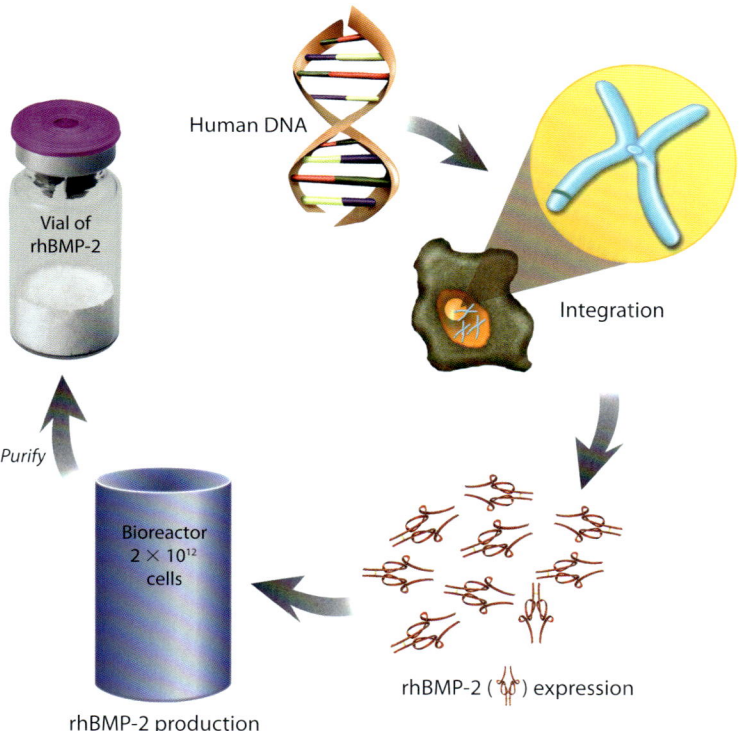

Because production cells can multiply further, a small number of cells become millions and millions, if allowed to incubate under the right conditions. Samples from the cell bank can be expanded for any future rhBMP-2 production. When production of rhBMP-2 is desired, a vial of rhBMP-2 production cells is thawed and placed in a flask containing cell culture medium. The medium contains all of the nutrients that the production cells need to multiply and to produce rhBMP-2. The cells are incubated for a period of time as the population expands. When the cell number is sufficient, the production cells are transferred to computer-controlled bioreactors, where large-scale production of rhBMP-2 begins. The production cells continue to grow, multiply, and secrete rhBMP-2 into the cell culture medium in which the production cells are suspended.

Periodically during production, a portion of the culture medium containing both rhBMP-2 and production cells is removed. The cells are separated from the rhBMP-2 through a filtration process and discarded. The solution then contains rhBMP-2, along with components of the culture medium and other proteins made naturally by the production cells. This solution is subjected to a series of steps to purify the rhBMP-2. The solution is passed through several different chromatography columns to separate rhBMP-2 from other proteins. The chromatography steps are followed by numerous filtration procedures, including a filter sterilization step. Quality control testing is performed throughout the rhBMP-2 production process to ensure the safety, quality, and purity of the material at each step. The result of this production process is a very pure ($>98\%$) solution of rhBMP-2. This rhBMP-2 solution is used to prepare individual protein vials containing freeze-dried rhBMP-2. The final product in the vial is simply reconstituted with sterile water for injection, producing a rhBMP-2 solution that is ready to be added to a carrier matrix and implanted at the site of application.

Safety of rhBMP-2

The safety of the rhBMP-2 protein has been evaluated in a series of studies.[3-24] These studies, discussed in the following sections, include toxicology studies, effects on reproduction, biocompatibility testing, pharmacokinetic studies, and tests of tumor cell growth potentiation. All of the preclinical studies performed to date indicate that rhBMP-2 is safe for clinical use in spinal fusion procedures.

When rhBMP-2 is placed on an absorbable collagen sponge (rhBMP-2/ACS) and implanted, rhBMP-2 is gradually released from the ACS matrix. The rhBMP-2/ACS combination maintains the local concentration of rhBMP-2 at the implantation site for a period long enough to induce new bone formation at that site. The released rhBMP-2 may also enter the bloodstream and potentially travel to sites far removed from the original implantation site. For this reason, intravenous and implant toxicity studies of rhBMP-2 have been performed. Acute toxicity studies were performed to assess whether adverse effects would result from systemic exposure to rhBMP-2 from a single bolus. A single intravenous dose of rhBMP-2 was administered to Sprague-Dawley rats and beagle dogs. Subchronic toxicity studies were also performed in the same species to determine the effects of multiple low-dose exposures to rhBMP-2.

Acute Toxicity Studies

In the acute toxicity study of rhBMP-2 in Sprague-Dawley rats, animals received a single intravenous bolus of one of five solutions.[3] The solutions included normal saline solution, a histidine/arginine vehicle, and three different doses of rhBMP-2 (0.053, 0.160, and 0.533 mg/kg). Fifteen animals of each sex received each treatment. Five animals per sex from each treatment group were sacrificed on days 2, 7, and 15. There were no treatment-related changes observed in this study. The no-toxic-effect level was 0.533 mg/kg.

A second single-dose intravenous study was performed in rats using a higher dose of rhBMP-2.[4] In this study, animals received a bolus of either buffer or rhBMP-2 in one of three doses (0.53, 1.6, or 5.3 mg/kg). There were 10 animals of each sex in each treatment group. One half of the animals in each treatment group were sacrificed on day 2, and the remaining animals were sacrificed on day 15.

There were no unscheduled deaths in either of the studies. Body weights, food consumption, clinical observations, and hematologic findings were unaffected by treatment. There were no treatment-related gross or histopathologic abnormalities other than the expected pharmacologic responses to rhBMP-2 at injection sites. Slight-to-moderate chondrogenesis at the site of injection was observed at the 0.53 mg/kg (one animal) and 5.3 mg/kg dosages (five animals). The no-toxic-effect level was 5.3 mg/kg. These changes represent the expected pharmacologic effect of rhBMP-2 and are toxicologically insignificant.

A similar study was performed in beagle dogs.[5] The treatment groups were the same as in the second Sprague-Dawley rat study (buffer, 0.53, 1.6, or 5.3 mg/kg rhBMP-2). Each treatment group consisted of one male and one female dog. The dogs received a single intravenous bolus of the appropriate treatment and were sacrificed on day 15. There were no unscheduled deaths. Body weights, food consumption, clinical observations, hematologic findings, and clinical chemistry showed no treatment-related effects. There were no treatment-related gross or histopathologic abnormalities. As in the previous study, the no-toxic-effect dose was

5.3 mg/kg. The highest dose used in these studies would correspond to a dose of 361 mg of rhBMP-2 in a 150-pound human. Table 3-1 summarizes the results of the acute toxicity studies.

Table 3-1

Acute Toxicity Studies to Assess Safety of a Single Intravenous Dose of rhBMP-2

Species/Strain	Number of Animals/ Sex/Group	Sacrifice Time	Treatment Groups	Relevant Findings
Rat/Sprague-Dawley[3]	5/sex/time point	Days 2, 7, and 15	Saline solution Buffer 0.053 mg/kg rhBMP-2 0.160 mg/kg rhBMP-2 0.533 mg/kg rhBMP-2	No toxicity observed No-toxic-effect dose was 0.533 mg/kg intravenously
Rat/Sprague-Dawley[4]	5/sex/time point	Days 2 and 15	Buffer 0.53 mg/kg rhBMP-2 1.6 mg/kg rhBMP-2 5.3 mg/kg rhBMP-2	No treatment-related findings in animals sacrificed at day 2 Slight to mild dose-related chondrogenesis at injection sites No-toxic-effect dose was 5.3 mg/kg intravenously
Canine/beagle[5]	1/sex/time point	Day 15	Buffer 0.53 mg/kg rhBMP-2 1.6 mg/kg rhBMP-2 5.3 mg/kg rhBMP-2	No toxicity observed No-toxic-effect dose was 5.3 mg/kg intravenously

Subchronic Toxicity Studies

Repeated-dose subchronic toxicity studies were also performed in Sprague-Dawley rats and beagle dogs.[6,7] In these studies, animals received once-daily intravenous administration of rhBMP-2 or buffer for 28 days. Three different doses of rhBMP-2 were investigated (0.016, 0.05, and 0.16 mg/kg). Animals were sacrificed after 28 days.

In the Sprague-Dawley rat study,[6] 10 animals of each sex were administered either buffer or rhBMP-2 solution daily and sacrificed at the end of the 28-day study. An additional five animals per sex in the control and high-dose rhBMP-2 groups were administered daily injections for 28 days and then sacrificed after a 28-day dose-free recovery period. There were 10 unscheduled deaths in this study. Four rats were sacrificed during the last week of the study, because bone induction at the tail vein injection site prevented additional dosing. Four other animals died during blood sampling on day 28, and two were sacrificed because of other complications. These deaths were considered to be unrelated to treatment. There were no treatment-related hematologic, clinical chemistry, urinalysis, or organ weight findings. Random, non–test-article-related gross pathologic findings were observed across all groups. Treatment-related and dose-related histopathologic findings at the injection site included soft tissue thickening as well as cartilage and bone formation. These changes were considered to be related to the expected pharmacologic action of rhBMP-2 and not toxicologically significant. The no-toxic-effect dose was 0.16 mg/kg/day.

In the study performed using beagle dogs,[7] three animals per sex/group were administered either buffer or rhBMP-2 solution daily and sacrificed at the end of 28 days. An additional two animals per sex in the control and high-dose groups were retained for a 28-day dose-free recovery period. There were no mortalities in this study group. Dose-related perivascular fibroplasia was observed at the injection site in all rhBMP-2–treated animals. Slight-to-severe osseous metaplasia of the fibrous tissue surrounding the injection site was observed in some animals. These changes were the expected result from the pharmacologic activity of rhBMP-2 and were not considered to be toxicologically significant. The no-toxic-effect dose was 0.16 mg/kg/day. These studies are summarized in Table 3-2.

Table 3-2

Subchronic Toxicity Studies to Assess Safety of Multiple Intravenous Doses of rhBMP-2

Species/Strain	Number of Animals/ Sex/Group	Sacrifice Time	Treatment Groups	Relevant Findings
Rat/Sprague-Dawley[6]	10/sex with 5/sex additional in recovery group for control and high-dose groups	28 days	Saline solution Buffer 0.016 mg/kg rhBMP-2 0.05 mg/kg rhBMP-2 0.16 mg/kg rhBMP-2	Ten deaths unrelated to treatment Dose-related soft tissue thickening and cartilage formation at injection site No-toxic-effect dose was 0.16 mg/kg/day intravenously
Canine/beagle[7]	3/sex with 2/sex additional in recovery group for control and high-dose groups	28 days	Buffer 0.016 mg/kg rhBMP-2 0.05 mg/kg rhBMP-2 0.16 mg/kg rhBMP-2	Dose-related perivascular fibroplasias at injection site in all rhBMP-2–treated animals No-toxic-effect dose was 0.16 mg/kg/day

These systemic studies of rhBMP-2 are important in that they contribute to the comprehensive study of the toxicity of the rhBMP-2 protein. However, it should be noted that intravenous administration of rhBMP-2 solution either singly or in repeated doses is not consistent with the way in which this protein is used clinically.

Reproductive Effects Studies

Several tests were performed to determine the effects of rhBMP-2 on fertility, reproduction, and embryo-fetal and perinatal toxicity.[8-10]

A study to assess the effects of rhBMP-2 on fertility and general reproductive performance was undertaken in both male and female Sprague-Dawley rats[8] (Table 3-3). Rats received either a saline control or one of three intravenous doses of rhBMP-2 (as high as 0.16 mg/kg/day). Treatment was administered to female rats daily from 2 weeks before mating through day 7 of gestation and to male rats from 2 weeks before mating through day 14 of the female rat gestation period. To distinguish effects on male and female fertility individually, treated female rats were mated with untreated males and treated male rats were mated with untreated females.

All rats were evaluated daily for gross signs of reaction to treatment, body weight, and food consumption. Other measurements for female rats included pathologic examination, mean days to mating, corpora lutea count, number and position of the embryos, live/dead embryo count, fertility rate, preimplantation and postimplantation losses, and resorption count. Other measurements for male rats included histopathologic examination of the testes and assessment of sperm, including motility, count, and morphology. The rhBMP-2 treatment (at any doses tested) had no effect on either reproduction or fertility in male and female rats.

Table 3-3

Tests to Assess Effects of rhBMP-2 on Reproduction

Species/Strain	Number of Animals/ Sex/Group	Sacrifice Time	Treatment Groups	Relevant Findings
Rat/Sprague-Dawley[8]	8/sex/group	Day 14 of gestation	Saline solution Buffer 0.016 mg/kg/day rhBMP-2 0.05 mg/kg/day rhBMP-2 0.16 mg/kg/day rhBMP-2	Maternal and paternal mating performance and reproductive parameters not affected by treatment No-toxic-effect dose was 0.16 mg/kg/day intravenously
Rabbit/New Zealand white[9]	20/female/group	Day 29 of gestation	Saline solution Buffer 0.016 mg/kg/day rhBMP-2 0.05 mg/kg/day rhBMP-2 0.16 mg/kg/day rhBMP-2 0.5 mg/kg/day rhBMP-2 1.6 mg/kg/day rhBMP-2 (Injections days 6 to 18 of gestation)	No maternal toxicity, embryolethality, or gross fetal abnormalities No-toxic-effect dose was 1.6 mg/kg/day intravenously
Rat/Sprague-Dawley[10]	25/female/group	Day 20 of gestation	Saline solution Buffer 0.16 mg/kg/day rhBMP-2 0.5 mg/kg/day rhBMP-2 1.6 mg/kg/day rhBMP-2 (Injections days 6 to 17 of gestation)	No maternal toxicity, embryolethality, or gross fetal abnormalities No-toxic-effect dose was 1.6 mg/kg/day intravenously

Additional studies were performed to assess embryo/fetal and perinatal toxicity. These teratology studies were performed in New Zealand white rabbits and Sprague-Dawley rats.[9,10] Inseminated female rabbits received intravenous injections of a control buffer or one of three different doses of rhBMP-2 (up to 1.6 mg/kg/day).[9] Daily treatments were administered from day 6 to day 18 of gestation. The parameters examined included daily clinical examination, body weight, food consumption, gross pathology, histopathology, number of live and dead fetuses, resorption count, pregnancy rate, sex ratio, preimplantation and postimplantation losses, fetal weight, and gross fetal abnormalities. The results of this study showed that treatment of gravid rabbits with rhBMP-2 did not result in systemic maternal toxicity, embryolethality, or gross fetal abnormalities at dosages up to 1.6 mg/kg/day.

The same study was also performed in Sprague-Dawley rats using the same three rhBMP-2 dosages and daily injections from day 6 to day 17 of gestation.[10] There was no evidence of maternal toxicity, embryolethality, fetotoxicity, or teratogenicity associated with rhBMP-2 treatment of rats at doses up to 1.6 mg/kg/day.

Biodistribution and Metabolism Studies

Toxicology studies using intravenous administration of rhBMP-2 or implantation of rhBMP-2/ACS have demonstrated no toxic effects of rhBMP-2 at doses much higher than those anticipated in clinical application of rhBMP-2. As these studies were designed to examine one aspect (potential toxicity) of the safety profile of rhBMP-2, they did not examine the fate of the rhBMP-2 protein that was injected into the bloodstream or implanted on the ACS matrix. In order to assess the biodistribution of injected protein or implanted rhBMP-2, a series of animal studies using radiolabeled rhBMP-2 protein was performed (Fig. 3-2).

The first set of experiments examined the absorption, distribution, metabolism, and excretion of rhBMP-2 following intravenous administration. These studies (in rats and monkeys) allowed the evaluation of systemic exposure to rhBMP-2 and characterization of the pharmacokinetics of rhBMP-2 in blood.[11-15] The studies showed that the pharmacokinetic profile of systemic rhBMP-2 is biphasic, with a rapid initial phase followed by a slower terminal phase. The rapid initial decline of rhBMP-2 observed following intravenous dosing suggests rapid distribution of the protein from the blood to highly perfused organs.

Figure 3-2

Percent of rhBMP-2 dose detected in the blood of rats following intravenous injection. Studies have shown that rhBMP-2 is rapidly eliminated from systemic circulation following intravenous administration.

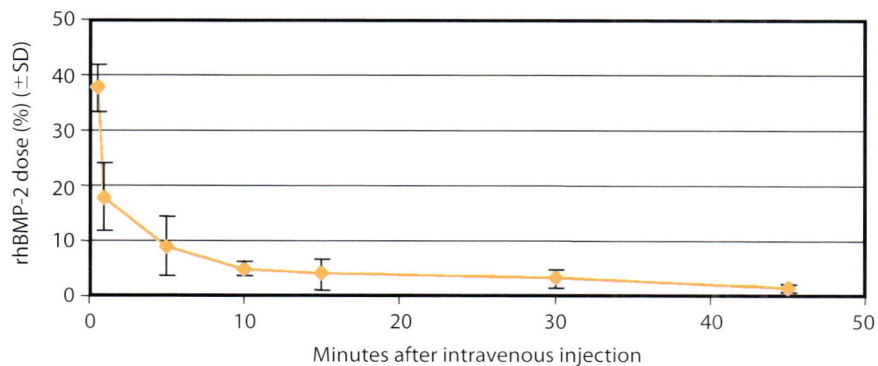

In a rat biodistribution study, 82.4% of the administered dose was found in the liver, kidney, spleen, and lung after only 1 minute.[15] After 5 minutes, 75% of the injected dose was located in the liver. Although distribution to these highly perfused organs was rapid, residence time in these organs was relatively short, with only 0.5% of the original dose detectable in these organs at 24 hours. These studies showed low exposure of rhBMP-2 in the circulation and short residence time in tissues and organs.

The available data suggest that rhBMP-2 is rapidly and extensively catabolized before being excreted via the renal pathway. In fact, 92% of the injected dose in rats was recovered as trichloroacetic acid (TCA)-soluble radioactivity in the urine within 24 hours of administration. Because TCA causes rhBMP-2 (and other proteins and peptides) to precipitate, these results suggest that rhBMP-2 is degraded by the body (into amino acids and small peptides) before being excreted in the urine.

Since systemic exposure to rhBMP-2 has not been detectable following rhBMP-2/ACS implantation in humans, pharmacokinetic parameters for humans have not been attainable. According to assumptions based on the available rat and primate data, an intravenous dose of 1 mg/kg in humans (which is much higher than the dose used in clinical applications) would be expected to yield a maximum rhBMP-2 concentration of around 0.02 µg/ml. This level is approximately 1000 times lower than a dose previously shown to be safe in preclinical acute toxicity studies. The results of the pharmacokinetic studies with rhBMP-2 delivered intravenously are summarized in Table 3-4.

Table 3-4

Pharmacokinetic Studies of rhBMP-2 Delivered Intravenously

Species/Strain	Number of Animals/ Group	Treatment Groups	Relevant Findings
PK Single Dose			
Rat/Sprague-Dawley[11]	3/group	0.43, 4.3, 43, 860 μg/kg/IV	Clearance of ^{125}I-rhBMP-2 rapid and biexponential (initial half-life = 0.8 min)
			92% of dose recovered in urine by 24 hr
Nonhuman primate[12]	3/group	4.9 μg/kg/IV	Clearance of ^{125}I-rhBMP-2 rapid and biexponential (initial half-life = 1 min)
Rat/Sprague-Dawley[13]	4/group	5.3 μg/kg/IV	Clearance of ^{125}I-rhBMP-2 rapid and biexponential (initial half-life = 0.6 min)
			Rapid localization to liver with metabolism and excretion into urine
Biodistribution			
Rat/Sprague-Dawley[14]	3/group	4.3 μg/kg/IV	Biphasic disposition with initial and terminal half-life of 0.8 and 31 min, respectively
			^{125}I-rhBMP-2 rapidly distributed to highly perfused tissues
Rat/Sprague-Dawley[15]	3/group	7.1 μg/kg/IV	Liver predominant site of ^{125}I-rhBMP-2 localization throughout the study
			1 min after dosing, 82.4% of dose recovered in liver, lung, kidney, and spleen

IV, Intravenously.

Assessment of Carcinogenicity and Toxicity

Some journal articles have reported the presence of BMP-2 in a number of human neoplasms. It has been suggested that the neoplastic epithelial cells or other elements of the tumor produce BMPs. However, BMPs have not been demonstrated or suggested to play a role in the primary neoplastic process. Rather, BMPs produced by tumor cells may lead to bone induction within the tumor. rhBMP-2 is a locally acting growth and differentiation factor. As such, rhBMP-2 binds to cells with the proper receptors and activates different genetic responses, dependent on the type of cell bound. As a differentiation factor, rhBMP-2 would theoretically act as an antitumor agent by forcing neoplastic cells to differentiate into other cell types.

The ability of rhBMP-2 to potentiate or inhibit tumor cell proliferation was examined using *in vitro* assays.[16] It should be noted that the short local residence time, the rapid systemic clearance of rhBMP-2, and the low systemic exposure to rhBMP-2 should all lower the risks of systemic effects due to rhBMP-2 exposure. Therefore any effect of rhBMP-2 on tumor cell growth would be relevant only in regard to the site of rhBMP-2/ACS implantation.

The potential effects of rhBMP-2 on tumor cell line growth were assessed at several concentrations up to 1000 ng/ml.[16] Four different human osteosarcoma cell lines were unaffected by exposure to rhBMP-2. The growth of two human prostate carcinomas, two breast carcinomas, a tongue carcinoma, and a lung carcinoma cell line were all inhibited by rhBMP-2.

Another set of experiments was performed in which primary tumor cell isolates were exposed to rhBMP-2 (10, 100, or 1000 ng/ml) *in vitro* in a colony-forming assay.[17] In these experiments, rhBMP-2 did not potentiate the growth in any of 65 isolates and significantly inhibited the growth of 16 of the 65 specimens. The tumor isolates were collected from ovarian carcinoma, breast carcinoma, non-small cell lung carcinoma, melanoma, and hepatoma. Other investigators have examined the effects of rhBMP-2 on tumor cell growth *in vitro*.[18-24] Two of these studies showed the possibility of stimulation of cell growth depending on the type of carcinoma and the culture conditions used. Ide[23] reported that rhBMP-2 could inhibit or stimulate the growth of prostate carcinoma cells depending on the culture media used. Kleeff[24] showed that rhBMP-2 could stimulate, inhibit, or have no effect on the growth of pancreatic tumor cell lines *in vitro* under starvation growth conditions.

In conclusion, there has been no evidence to suggest a causal role for rhBMP-2 in tumor formation and little evidence of the potential for rhBMP-2 to increase the growth rate of tumor cells. In addition, the lack of systemic exposure prevents rhBMP-2 from having any influence on tumor cells at any site other than the site of implantation. Because a tumor cell growth potentiating effect cannot be completely ruled out, it is recommended that the rhBMP-2/ACS implant not be implanted into a site of known tumor formation, in the vicinity of a resected or extant tumor, in patients with an active malignancy, or in patients undergoing treatment for a malignancy.

Role of Carrier

One of the greatest hurdles in the development of bone graft substitutes that contain BMPs has been the identification of an effective carrier for the BMP protein. The importance of the carrier was underestimated in the early development of BMPs. It was later determined that the carrier served three very important functions (Fig. 3-3):
1. Acts as a three-dimensional space occupier in an area where new bone is desired (i.e., space maintenance)
2. Maintains a critical level of BMP at the site of implantation for the desired period of time by slowly releasing the adsorbed rhBMP-2 and maintaining the threshold concentration
3. Acts as a scaffold for new bone deposition and vascularization

Rationale and Criteria for rhBMP-2 Carriers

The ideal carrier for BMP should have the following characteristics:
- Biocompatibility
- BMP-binding capacity
- Handling ease during surgery
- BMP release over an adequate period of time
- Space maintenance for new bone deposition
- Osteoconductive surface for osteoid deposition
- Ability to resorb at a rate compatible with new bone formation and remodeling

Figure 3-3

The rhBMP-2 carrier should serve three important functions: maintain space, maintain critical concentration of rhBMP-2, and act as scaffold for new bone.

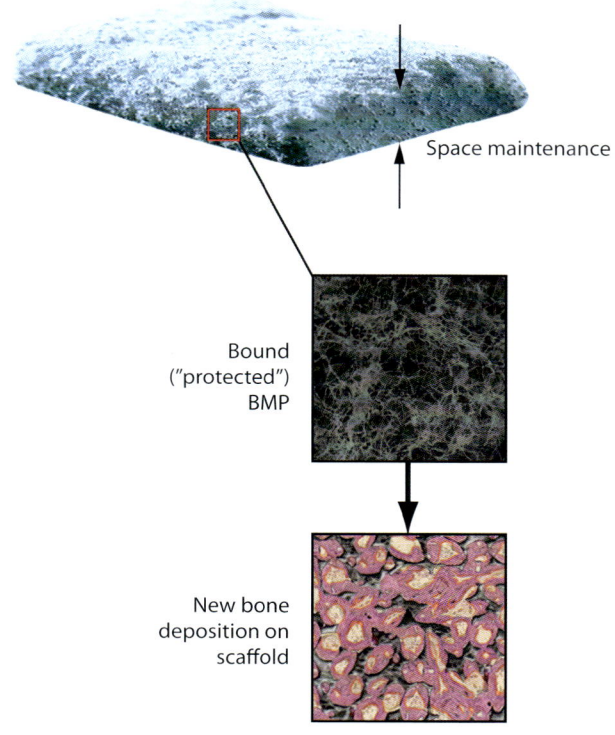

The only definitive method of determining the effectiveness of a carrier is through preclinical research, which is a long, iterative process taking several years of investigation. As illustrated in Fig. 3-4, the ideal carrier undergoes resorption at a rate that matches the rate of new bone formation. In other words, as osteoid or new bone is deposited on the carrier scaffold, the carrier scaffold undergoes resorption, leaving behind only the new bone. If the carrier resorbs before osteoid deposition, inadequate bone formation results.

Further complicating the identification of the ideal carrier is the fact that the rate of bone formation is species dependent. Therefore preclinical work had to be carried out in a higher-order species (i.e., nonhuman primates) with a relatively slow rate of bone formation similar to that of humans (Fig. 3-5). The carrier had to have a slow enough resorption profile to match the slow rate of new bone formation in higher-order species to better ensure its effectiveness in humans. Lower-order animal studies (e.g., rodents and canines) would produce misleading results that do not directly translate to human clinical use.

One additional complicating factor in this research is the finding that the concentration of BMP has an effect on the degradation rate of the carrier. Consequently, prior data on the resorption profile of different biomaterials that were potential carrier candidates had to be evaluated in preclinical studies in combination with BMP to reestablish their resorption profile in the presence of BMP.

In summary, the following three issues must be taken into account in the identification and development of carriers for BMP:
1. Evaluation of new carriers must be developed through preclinical research.
2. Preclinical research needs to be carried out in higher-order species.
3. A carrier material's resorption profile is dependent on BMP concentration.

Figure 3-4

The rate of new bone deposition must be matched to the resorption rate. Results from a rat study.

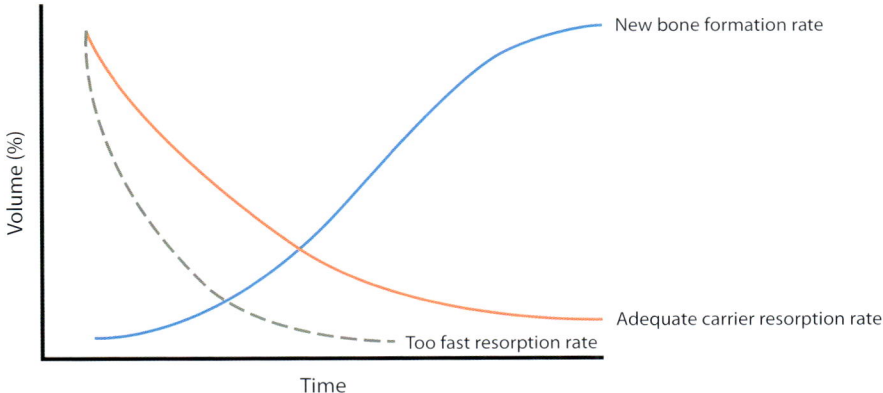

 Figure 3-5

The rate of new bone deposition is different in higher-order species compared with lower order. The carrier resorption rate versus bone deposition is determined experimentally in preclinical research.

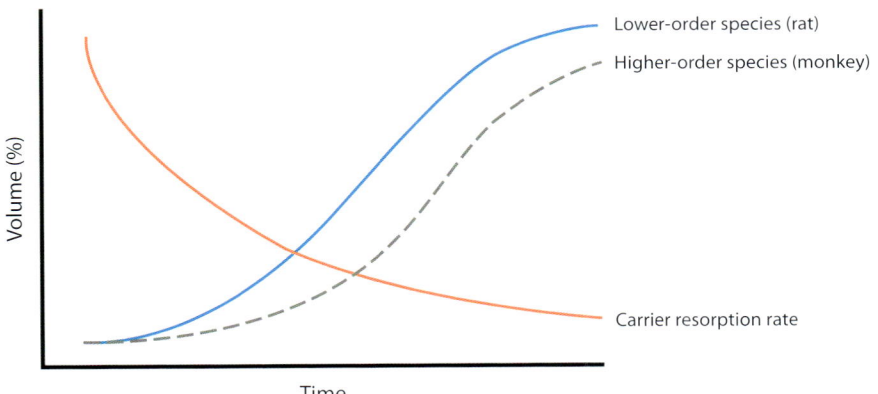

Frequently Asked Questions

What is the overall safety profile of rhBMP-2?

The protein has been tested in dozens of preclinical (animal) safety studies. These studies show that, even at doses that are thousands of times higher than the expected human exposures, rhBMP-2 has an excellent safety profile.

How is rhBMP-2 excreted from the body? How long is it present in the body?

rhBMP-2 is only present at the implant site for 3 to 4 weeks and is cleared from the blood by the liver and excreted via the urine.

What is the concern regarding rhBMP-2 and cancers?

The patient population in the clinical studies had the same incidence rate for cancers whether rhBMP-2/ACS or autograft was used. However, because BMPs, among many other proteins, can be found in some tumors, and because ossification of some tumors occurs, a few investigators have suggested using it as a diagnostic tool. In general, research has demonstrated that rhBMP-2 either has no impact on cancer cell line growth or human tumors implanted in mice, or it decreases the growth. When increased growth occurred (in three cases), the cell culture environment lacked serum, making the results clinically irrelevant. Some researchers have suggested that rhBMP-2 could be an anticancer therapeutic, as it was inhibitory to a number of cell lines, but the response is not considered strong enough for investigation at this time.

What about the potential for fetal problems in patients having used rhBMP-2?

The BMP family of proteins is involved in a number of events during fetal development. As they are so important, any deactivation of fetal BMP-2 would be very detrimental. Antibodies to rhBMP-2, if produced and able to cross the placenta, could deactivate fetal BMP-2.

Several studies were undertaken during the preclinical phase in both rodents and rabbits (see Table 3-3). No effect on any of the numerous parameters involved in pregnancy or fertility was seen.

Women of childbearing potential should be advised that antibody formation to rhBMP-2 or its influence on fetal development have not been assessed. In the clinical trial supporting the safety and effectiveness of the INFUSE® Bone Graft/LT-CAGE® Lumbar Tapered Fusion Device, 0.7% patients treated with INFUSE® Bone Graft and 0.8% patients treated with autograft bone developed antibodies to rhBMP-2.[25] The effect on the unborn fetus of maternal antibodies to rhBMP-2, which might be present for several months following device implantation, is unknown. Additionally, it is unknown whether fetal expression of BMP-2 could re-expose mothers who were previously antibody positive, thereby eliciting a more powerful immune response to BMP-2 with adverse consequences for the fetus. Studies in genetically altered mice indicate that BMP-2 is critical to fetal development and that lack of BMP-2 activity, as might be induced by antibody formation, may cause neonatal death or birth defects. Women of childbearing potential should be advised to not become pregnant for one year following treatment with INFUSE® Bone Graft.

REFERENCES

1. Wang EA, Rosen V, Cordes P, et al. Purification and characterization of other distinct bone-inducing factors. Proc Natl Acad Sci USA 85:9484-9488, 1988.
2. Wozney JM, Rosen V, Celeste AJ, et al. Novel regulators of bone formation: Molecular clones and activities. Science 242:1528-1534, 1988.
3. Internal document. Single-Dose Toxicity Study, GI 52585.
4. Internal document. Single-Dose Toxicity Study, GI 53950.
5. Internal document. Single-Dose Toxicity Study, GI 52586.
6. Internal document. Subchronic Toxicity Study, GI 52587.
7. Internal document. Subchronic Toxicity Study, GI Report 52588.
8. Internal document. Reproductive Function, GI 95851.
9. Internal document. Teratology Study, GI 95476.
10. Internal document. Teratology Study, GI 95477.
11. Internal document. Distribution Study, GI Report PB-034-91.
12. Internal document. Distribution Study, GI Report PB-024-92.
13. Internal document. Distribution Study, GI Report PB-009-94.
14. Internal document. Distribution Study, GI Report PB-035-91.
15. Internal document. Distribution Study, GI Report PS-008-94.
16. Internal document. Osteosarcoma Study, GI Report PB-040-91.
17. Soda H, Raymond E, Sharma S, et al. Antiproliferative effects of recombinant human bone morphogenetic protein-2 on human tumor colony-forming units. Anticancer Drugs 9:327-331, 1998.
18. Arnold SF, Tims E, McCrath BE. Identification of bone morphogenetic proteins and their receptors in human breast cancer cell lines: Importance of BMP2. Cytokine 11:1031-1037, 1999.
19. Hjertner O, Hjorth-Hansen H, Borset M, et al. Bone morphogenetic protein-4 inhibits proliferation and induces apoptosis of multiple myeloma cells. Blood 97:516-522, 2001.
20. Nozaki K, Kadosawa T, Nishimura R, et al. 1,25-Dihydroxyvitamin D3, recombinant human transforming growth factor-beta 1, and recombinant human bone morphogenetic protein-2 induce in vitro differentiation of canine osteosarcoma cells. J Vet Med Sci 61:649-656, 1999.
21. Yokouchi Y, Sakiyama J, Kameda T, et al. BMP-2/-4 mediate programmed cell death in chicken limb buds. Development 122:3725-3734, 1996.
22. Yamato K, Hashimoto S, Okahashi N, et al. Dissociation of bone morphogenetic protein-mediated growth arrest and apoptosis of mouse B cells by HPV-16 E6/E7. Exp Cell Res 257:198-205, 2000.

23. Ide H, Yoshida T, Matsumoto N, et al. Growth regulation of human prostate cancer cells by bone morphogenetic protein-2. Cancer Res 57:5022-5027, 1997.
24. Kleeff J, Maruyama H, Ishiwata T, et al. Bone morphogenetic protein-2 exerts diverse effects on cell growth in vitro and is expressed in human pancreatic cancer in vivo. Gastroenterology 116:1202-1216, 1999.
25. Burkus JK, Gornet MF, Dickman CA, et al. Anterior lumbar interbody fusion using rhBMP-2 with tapered interbody cages. J Spinal Disord Tech 15:337-349, 2002.

CHAPTER 4

rhBMP-2 and ACS

Selection of ACS as rhBMP-2 Carrier

One of the optimal rhBMP-2 carriers that has been identified is the type I bovine absorbable collagen sponge (ACS). The ACS has been commercially available as an absorbable hemostatic agent since 1981 (Helistat®, Integra Life Sciences, Plainsboro, NJ) (Fig. 4-1). The ACS is made of a natural fibrillar collagen material. Because gelatin undergoes relatively rapid degradation in contrast to fibrillar collagen, it is not a good carrier for BMP. Resorption of the gelatin occurs too soon after implantation and before it can act as a scaffold for new bone formation.

Once implanted, the ACS undergoes resorption over a 4- to 12-week period via cell-mediated degradation by the macrophages.[1,2] Collagen provides a favorable surface for cell attachment during early osteoid for-

 Figure 4-1

The reconstituted rhBMP-2 is evenly deposited on the collagen sponge and readily adsorbed onto the sponge.

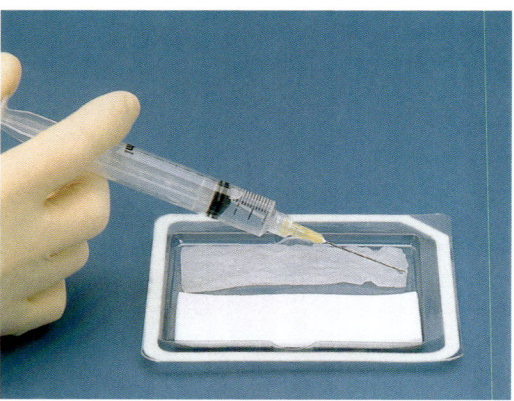

mation and then undergoes resorption. As part of the selection process, more than 100 different carriers were screened before the ACS was chosen. The collagen sponge appears to possess all the properties of an ideal carrier for BMP.

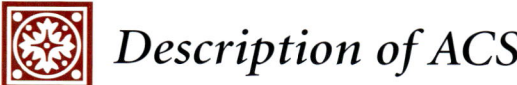 Description of ACS

The absorbable collagen sponge is derived from the Achilles tendon of steers at the beginning of beef production. The Achilles tendon is harvested before the butchering of the steer occurs to prevent contamination from neural tissue. The tendons are harvested in the United States from USDA-cleared food-grade herds.

The tendon tissue is virtually avascular and is the first tissue to be harvested, which reduces the risk of infection or contamination. After harvesting, the tendon is treated extensively with alkali solutions to become the spongelike material that has been used for several decades in surgical hemostasis. After the collagen is formed into a sponge, the material is sterilized with ethylene oxide. The sponge material is extensively tested for a large number of possible viral contaminants to ensure that it is safe for clinical use.

The type I bovine collagen in the ACS sponge has similarities in chemical structure to the type I collagen in human bodies, which could theoretically cause human antibody production against human type I collagen. No such problem has surfaced during the 20 years of Helistat® use. The formation of bovine collagen antibodies in response to the implantation of rhBMP-2/ACS was studied as part of human clinical trials and will be discussed in Chapter 6.

Characterization of rhBMP-2 and ACS Binding

rhBMP-2 binds naturally to the ACS. This binding offers the advantages of applying the rhBMP-2-soaked collagen sponge surgically and minimizing the loss of rhBMP-2 during handling. To ensure sufficient binding of rhBMP-2 to the ACS, a minimum of 15 minutes soaking time is recommended. The rhBMP-2–soaked sponge should be used within 2 hours of applying the rhBMP-2 to the ACS. This last limitation was established as a precaution to prevent the sponge from drying out.

The binding of rhBMP-2 to the ACS has been studied using two methods: (1) by removing all of the fluid from the sponge with centrifugation and measuring the rhBMP-2 remaining in the dry sponge, and (2) by measuring the rhBMP-2 in the fluid released with normal intraoperative handling of the wet ACS. Each of these experiments was conducted after the sponge soaked in rhBMP-2 solution for either 15 or 120 minutes. After 15 minutes of soaking, approximately 52% of the applied rhBMP-2 remained in the dry collagen sponge after centrifugation. A longer soaking time of 120 minutes increased the binding of rhBMP-2 to the ACS to 72% (Fig. 4-2). The amount of rhBMP-2 remaining in the wet ACS under normal handling conditions, estimated from the concentration in expressed fluid, was found to be 95% after 15 minutes of soaking and increased to 97% after 120 minutes.[3] These studies verified that the ACS is effective as a carrier that incorporates and delivers rhBMP-2 to the site of application. The studies also verified that loss of rhBMP-2 during normal handling is minimal.

Figure 4-2

Binding of rhBMP-2 to the ACS carrier at 15 and 120 minutes. The percentage of rhBMP-2 remaining in a dry sponge after all the fluid has been removed by centrifugation is compared with the percentage of rhBMP-2 remaining in a wet sponge after normal intraoperative handling.

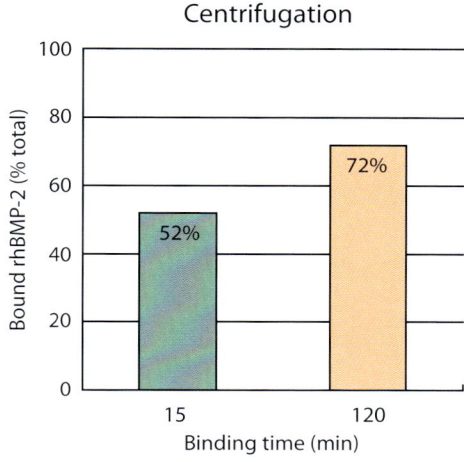

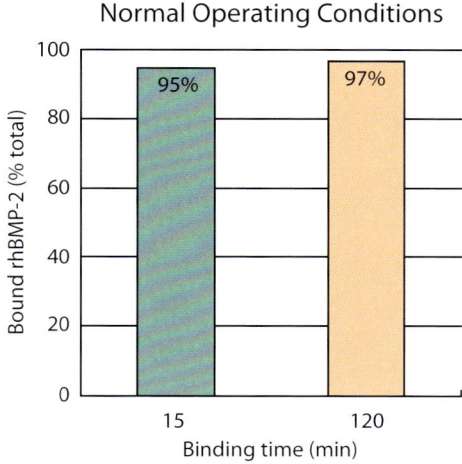

The *in vivo* release of rhBMP-2 from the ACS after implantation has been studied using radiolabeled rhBMP-2. The local residence time of rhBMP-2 when applied to the ACS has been assessed following subcutaneous (SC) implantation in rats and implantation at orthotopic sites in rats and rabbits. The results from all 3 models were similar. In the rat femoral onlay model, ^{125}I-rhBMP-2 was slowly released from the implant site with a mean residence time of approximately 8 days (Fig. 4-3).[4] It was determined that the half-life of rhBMP-2 was approximately 2 days and rhBMP-2 was undetectable after 3 weeks.

The relative retention of rhBMP-2 has been shown to be unaffected by the concentration of rhBMP-2 administered (between 0.8 and 2.0 mg/cc). The amount of rhBMP-2 incorporated into the ACS (a measure of the binding of rhBMP-2 to the sponge before implantation) had a minimal

Figure 4-3

The local residence time of rhBMP-2 when applied to the ACS was assessed following implantation at orthotopic sites. Amount of rhBMP-2 at the implant site (as a percentage of the original dose) is shown over time following surgical administration of the rhBMP-2/ACS in rats.

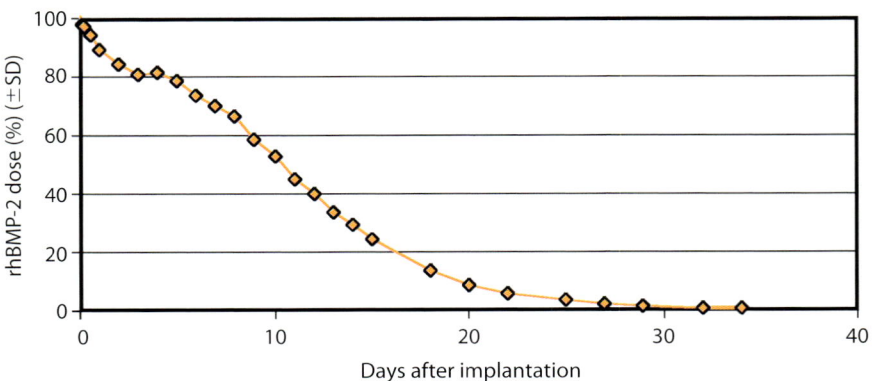

effect on rhBMP-2 retention *in vivo*, and no effect on the rate of release of rhBMP-2 into serum *in vitro*. These results suggest that the release of rhBMP-2 *in vivo* is independent of the binding of rhBMP-2 to the sponge *in vitro* and may occur via a diffusion-controlled release mechanism.

Safety of rhBMP-2/ACS

In addition to the safety studies for rhBMP-2 alone, the rhBMP-2/ACS combination product has undergone a number of safety assessments. These studies assessed toxicology, biocompatibility, and biodistribution. In addition, chronic toxicity studies were performed to examine the effects of long-term exposure to rhBMP-2/ACS. In these studies, rhBMP-2/ACS was implanted at bony sites to model some of the clinical uses of the product. All of the preclinical studies performed to date indicate that rhBMP-2 by itself and in combination with the ACS is safe for clinical use in spinal fusion procedures.

Chronic Toxicity Studies

The chronic toxicity of rhBMP-2/ACS was assessed in beagle dogs and Sprague-Dawley rats[5,6] (Table 4-1). In these studies rhBMP-2 was applied to an ACS matrix and implanted into the animals in either a mandibular/maxillofacial inlay model (dogs) or a femoral onlay model (rats). This method of application is consistent with some aspects of the clinical use of rhBMP-2/ACS.

Table 4-1

Chronic Toxicity Studies to Assess Safety of Implanted rhBMP-2/ACS

Species/Strain	Number of Animals/ Sex/Group	Sacrifice Time	Treatment Groups	Relevant Findings
Canine/ beagle[5]	2/sex/time point	3 and 6 months	Buffer 0.078 mg/kg/ ACS 0.312 mg/kg/ ACS 0.781 mg/kg/ ACS	No effects of treatment on clinical, hematologic, or clinical chemistry studies Dose-related post-surgical swelling reached a maximum 1-2 weeks after surgery Implant site tissue responses were the expected pharmacologic response to rhBMP-2/ACS and not toxicologically significant No-toxic-effect dose was 0.781 mg/kg
Rat/Sprague-Dawley[6]	10/sex/time point	1, 6, and 12 months	Buffer/ACS 0.04 mg/kg/ ACS 0.3 mg/kg/ ACS 1.6 mg/kg/ ACS	Slight increase in incidence of surgical site swelling at 1.6 mg/kg Dose-related incidence of bone formation at implant site No toxicity at any dose No-toxic-effect dose was 1.6 mg/kg

In the mandibular/maxillofacial inlay study, beagle dogs received either ACS matrix alone or rhBMP-2/ACS (0.078, 0.312, and 0.781 mg/kg) implanted bilaterally in the mandible and zygoma.[5] Two animals per sex were sacrificed at 3 months and another two per sex were sacrificed 6 months after implantation. Daily clinical examinations were performed on all animals, including an examination of the implant site, body weight, and food consumption. Additional evaluations included ophthalmoscopy, ECG, blood pressure measurement, hematologic studies, clinical chemistry analysis, urinalysis, and measurement of antibody response to rhBMP-2 and bovine collagen. Each animal underwent gross examination at sacrifice, and the rhBMP-2/ACS implant site tissues were retained for histopathologic examination.

There were no treatment-related adverse systemic effects. Dose-related increases in postsurgical swelling reached a maximum 1 to 2 weeks after surgery. Histologic evaluation of the implant sites revealed dose-related fibrocellular tissue and/or new bone formation within and around the implant sites in the rhBMP-2–treated groups. The only implant tissue responses were the expected pharmacologic response to rhBMP-2/ACS and were not toxicologically relevant. No antibody response to bovine collagen occurred. A transient low-titer antibody response to rhBMP-2 was observed in 15 of 24 treated animals. No systemic toxicity was observed at any dose level, and the no-toxic-effect dose was 0.78 mg/kg.

The safety of rhBMP-2/ACS was also evaluated in a Sprague-Dawley rat femoral onlay model.[6] In this study there were four groups of 30 animals per sex, with 10 animals per sex sacrificed at each time point (1, 6, and 12 months). A control and three different groups receiving rhBMP-2 on the ACS matrix were used in this study (0.04, 0.3, and 1.6 mg/kg). Systemic toxicity parameters assessed included clinical observations, body weights, food consumption, ophthalmologic examinations, hematologic findings, clinical chemistry analyses, urinalysis, and full gross and histopathologic evaluations. Serum was also collected for analysis of antibody titers to rhBMP-2 or bovine collagen.

There were no treatment-related adverse effects on any parameters assessed. No measurable antibody response in any animal was found. Treatment-related swellings were observed at the implant sites. These observations correlated to periosteal new bone formation. When the 26-week and 52-week sacrifices were compared with the 4-week samples, there appeared to be normal remodeling of the new bone. No toxicity was associated with rhBMP-2/ACS during the 52-week duration of the study. The no-toxic-effect dose was 1.6 mg/kg.

Standard Biocompatibility Tests

An additional set of studies was performed on rhBMP-2/ACS according to the FDA Tripartite Biocompatibility Guidelines.[7] An intracutaneous toxicity study[8] showed no evidence of significant irritation or toxicity in response to rhBMP-2/ACS extracts. Additionally, no systemic toxicity was associated with IV or intraperitoneal exposure to rhBMP-2/ACS extracts.[9] Other studies indicated that rhBMP-2/ACS extracts caused no cell lysis or toxicity,[10,11] no hemolysis,[12] no mutagenesis,[13] and no signs of sensitization.[14] In a surgical muscle implantation study,[15-18] the rhBMP-2/ACS was graded as a slight irritant because of a hard granular formation around the test site. Histologic evaluation revealed the formation to be new bone at the implant site that is consistent with the known pharmacologic action of rhBMP-2. The results of these biocompatibility tests of rhBMP-2/ACS are summarized in Table 4-2.

Table 4-2

Studies to Assess Biocompatibility of rhBMP-2/ACS According to FDA Tripartite Biocompatibility Guidelines

Study Type	Number of Animals/Sex/Group	Relevant Findings
Intracutaneous toxicity[8]	2/sex	No evidence of significant irritation or toxicity
Systemic toxicity[9]	20/sex	Not considered systemically toxic
Cytotoxicity/*in vitro*[10,11]	NA	No evidence of cell lysis or toxicity
In vitro hemolysis[12]	1	Not considered hemolytic
Ames *in vitro* mutagenicity study[13]	NA	Not considered mutagenic
Delayed contact sensitization[14]	15 female	No evidence of sensitization
Surgical muscle implantation study[15-18]	2	Considered to be trace to mild irritants after implantation in muscle

NA, Data not available.

Biodistribution Studies

Biodistribution assays with rhBMP-2/ACS were also performed using ^{125}I-labeled rhBMP-2.[4,19] The rhBMP-2/ACS was implanted in either a rat femoral onlay model or a rat subcutaneous ectopic implant model. The blood concentration of rhBMP-2 and the retention of rhBMP-2 by the ACS were determined by measuring the amount of radioactivity in blood samples or at the implant site. In the rat femoral onlay model, the mean residence time of rhBMP-2 was 78 days[4] (see Fig. 4-3). The maximum level of rhBMP-2 detected in the circulation was 0.1% of the implanted dose and was observed at the 6-hour time point.

In the study using a rat ectopic implant model, the mean residence time ranged from 3.6 to 4.6 days.[19] In this model, the retention kinetics of rhBMP-2 were independent of rhBMP-2 concentration over a large concentration range (0.08 to 2.0 mg/cc). The results of biodistribution studies of rhBMP-2/ACS are summarized in Table 4-3.

Table 4-3

Pharmacokinetic Studies of Implanted rhBMP-2/ACS

Species/Strain	Number of Animals/Sex/Group	Treatment Groups (mg/cc)/Route	Relevant Findings
Femoral Onlay			
Rat/Long Evans[4]	9/group	0.4 (implant)	Low system availability
			Mean residence time of rhBMP-2 estimated to be 7.8 days
Ectopic Implant			
Rat/Long Evans[19]	12/group	0.08	Retention profile biexponential over 14-day period
		0.40	No dependence on rhBMP-2 concentration over range used
		2.00 (implant)	Mean residence time ranged from 3.6 to 4.6 days

Mechanisms and Timing of rhBMP-2/ACS–Induced Bone Formation

The timing of bone formation when using rhBMP-2/ACS as a bone graft substitute in rhesus monkeys was assessed in a study by Boden et al.[20] CTs and radiographs obtained at 12 weeks after implantation demonstrate that dose has an impact on the speed of bone induction. The bone graft implanted was either 0.75 mg/cc or 1.5 mg/cc rhBMP-2/ACS. The use of the sponge alone also determined that no spontaneous healing occurred. The higher concentration delivered radiographic arthrodesis more rapidly than the lower dose, whereas the lower dose, although effective, produced a slower result. A complete bony bridge was seen anteriorly in all three of the rhBMP-2 monkeys that were treated with the 1.5 mg/cc concentration. A partial bridge was observed in 1 of the autograft control animals, and in 1 of the 2 treated with the lower dose. The histological assessment "demonstrated normal, mature trabecular bone surrounding and growing through the cages in the animals with rhBMP-2 and correlated with the sagittal CT scan findings." At 24 weeks, there was no appreciable difference in the amount of bone formation between low and high dose animals. In animal models, the timing of rhBMP-2-induced fusion is more rapid than that achieved with autograft.

In an elegantly designed rabbit gene expression study, Morone et al[21] observed the genetic expression of several products that are instrumental in bone development. The autograft subjects were compared with rabbits treated with rhBMP-2–soaked autograft bone. Data points for gene expression in autograft and autograft/rhBMP-2–treated rabbits were gathered at 2 and 4 days and 1, 2, 3, 4, 5, 6, and 10 weeks and compared with baseline iliac crest bone. In the animals receiving autograft alone, gene expression in the central zone of the fusion mass lagged 1 to 2 weeks behind that of the two outer zones and correlated with a central lag effect seen previously in histologic healing sequences. In the outer zones, increased BMP-2 expression peaked in weeks 3 and 4 for a 40-fold increase. In the rhBMP-2–treated animals, there was a dramatic impact on gene expression during the fusion process. This was especially notable for BMP-6, although expression of other bone-related genes was seen earlier and at higher levels than in autograft alone. The lag effect in the central zone was minimized.

Frequently Asked Questions

What is the clinical use history of ACS?

The ACS was FDA-approved in 1981 after a PMA application and has been used clinically since then.

Discuss the importance of the soaking time for the rhBMP-2 solution with the sponge.

The ACS is uniformly wetted after 15 minutes of soaking time. This is the minimum soaking time recommended to ensure sufficient rhBMP-2 binding. Based on the animal studies, a 60-minute soaking time does not alter the positive results obtained with a 15-minute soaking time. Under normal handling conditions, 95% of the rhBMP-2 is retained within the wet ACS carrier after 15 minutes. The sponge should be used within 2 hours of applying the rhBMP-2.

Is the collagen sponge left in the body after the surgical procedure is completed?

Yes, the collagen sponge allows the protein to stay in place long enough to exert the osteoinductive activity. The sponge is subsequently resorbed by the body. Histology from animal models suggests that the collagen sponge is resorbed in 4 to 12 weeks.[1,2]

The ACS is made of bovine collagen. Are there any issues with BSE and ACS?

There are no bovine spongiform encephalitis (BSE) or transmissible spongiform encephalitis (TSE) issues with the ACS. The sponge has been used clinically for 20 years and has been the subject of three IDEs. There have been no problems. The Achilles tendon is removed from food-grade steers before butchering without contamination with neural tissue.

What is the viral safety of the sponge and the rhBMP-2?

The ACS is extensively tested to determine viral contamination. It is also terminally sterilized by ethylene oxide. The rhBMP-2 is purified through column chromatography at production and tested for presence of viral contamination before release. The rhBMP-2 solution is terminally sterilized by filtration.

Are there any stability (sterility) issues with ACS?

The commercial product is stored at room temperature. There are no issues with sterility at room temperature. There have been no sterility issues for the length of the 20-year clinical use of the ACS.

What are the antibody or autoimmune issues with the ACS?

The sponge is made of bovine type I collagen. As type I collagen also exists in the human body, autoimmune responses from use of the ACS would probably take the form of an anti-collagen response. If there is a clinically relevant antibody response to bovine collagen, the potential exists for an antibody response to human collagen. In the pivotal clinical trial using INFUSE® Bone Graft /LT-CAGE® Device,[22] all patients receiving the ACS with rhBMP-2 were tested for bovine collagen antibody. Of patients receiving INFUSE® Bone Graft, 12.6% developed an antibody response to bovine type I collagen, compared with 11.8% in the ICBG control group.[23] Positive response patients were tested for human collagen antibody. There were no positive results for human collagen antibody in the patients that evidenced a bovine collagen response. There were also no adverse clinical outcomes where there was a bovine antibody response.

Moreover, the presence of antibodies to rhBMP-2 was not associated with immune-mediated adverse events such as allergic reactions. The neutralizing capacity of antibodies to rhBMP-2 is not known.

It should be noted that the incidence of antibody detection is highly dependent on the sensitivity and specificity of the assay. Additionally, the incidence of antibody detection may be influenced by several factors including sample handling, concomitant medications and underlying disease. For these reasons, comparison of the incidence of antibodies to the INFUSE® Bone Graft component with the incidence of antibodies to other products may be misleading.[24]

What is the resorption rate of the ACS?

Histology from animal models suggests that the collagen sponge is resorbed in 4 to 12 weeks.[1,2]

Discuss the quality of bone formed when using rhBMP-2.

Animal explant studies give complete confidence that real bone (not simply calcified material) is formed. This is true by 4 weeks in rabbits and by 16 to 24 weeks in rhesus monkeys. In addition, bone harvested at the time of dental implant placement in a human clinical study of sinus floor augmentation with rhBMP-2/ACS has shown that the new bone induced by rhBMP-2/ACS has the appearance of healthy trabecular bone.[25]

Remodeling of the trabecular bone induced by rhBMP-2/ACS occurs in a manner that is consistent with the biomechanical forces placed on it. Radiographic, biomechanical, and histologic evaluation of the induced bone indicates that it functions biologically and biomechanically as native bone. Furthermore, preclinical studies have indicated that the bone induced by rhBMP-2/ACS can repair itself, if fractured, in a manner indistinguishable from native bone healing.[26]

Is the sensitivity of CT scans specific for mature bone?

In a CT assessment of the fusion induced by rhBMP-2/ACS, Burkus et al[27] report an increase in bone density at 6-, 12-, and 24-month time points. The authors also note that new bone formation outside of the cages occurs more rapidly in rhBMP-2/ACS–treated patients than in autograft patients. The presence of dense bridging bone within the cage indicates the maturity of the bone.

Were there any clinical signs at the site of implantation (e.g., inflammation)?

There were no adverse effects or infection at the implantation site in the clinical studies that were related to rhBMP-2 and ACS.

REFERENCES

1. Internal document. GI Report BBA94073-11.
2. Internal document. GI Report BBA-94007.
3. Spector M, Zanella JM, Peckham SM, et al. Release of recombinant human bone morphogenetic protein-2 from absorbable collagen during the mechanical compression associated with its use for spinal fusion Transactions of the Orthopaedic Research Society Annual Meeting, 29:Paper 1140, San Francisco, 2004.
4. Internal document. Retention Kinetic Study, GI Report PS-009-94.
5. Internal document. Chronic Toxicity Study, GI 94014.
6. Internal document. Chronic Toxicity Study, GI 94105.
7. FDA Tripartite Biocompatibility Guidance, April 24, 1987 (G87-1). Food and Drug Administration website: *http://www.fda.gov/cdrh/g87-1.html*.
8. Internal document. Intracutaneous Study, GI TU013-800.
9. Internal document. Systemic Toxicity Study, GI T-12-500.
10. Internal document. Cytotoxicity Study, GI MG023-200.
11. Internal document. Cytotoxicity Study, GI MG030-110.
12. Internal document. Hemolysis Study, GI CB036-100.
13. Internal document. Mutagenesis Study, GI MG019-211.
14. Internal document. Sensitization Study, GI TA006-300.
15. Internal document. Muscle Implantation Study, GI TU019-814.
16. Internal document. Muscle Implantation Study, GI TU014-001.
17. Internal document. Muscle Implantation Study, GI TH035-800.
18. Internal document. Muscle Implantation Study, GI TH035-001.
19. Internal document. Recovery Study, GI Report BBA-95031.
20. Boden SD, Martin GJ Jr, Horton WC, et al. Laparoscopic anterior spinal arthrodesis with rhBMP-2 in a titanium interbody threaded cage. J Spinal Disord 11:95-101, 1998.
21. Morone MA, Boden SD, Hair G, et al. The Marshall R. Urist Young Investigator Award. Gene expression during autograft lumbar spine fusion and the effect of bone morphogenetic protein 2. Clin Orthop Relat Res 351:252-265, 1998.
22. Burkus JK, Gornet M, Dickman CA, et al. Anterior lumbar interbody fusion using rhBMP-2 with tapered interbody cages. J Spinal Disord Tech 15:337-349, 2002.
23. Summary of Safety And Effectiveness Data, PMA P000058. Food and Drug Administration website: *http://www.fda.gov/cdrh/pdf/P000058b.pdf*, p 37. Posted July 11, 2002.
24. Summary of Safety And Effectiveness Data, PMA P000058. Food and Drug Administration website: *http://www.fda.gov/cdrh/pdf/P000058b.pdf*, p 4. Posted July 11, 2002.

25. Boyne PJ, Marx RE, Nevins M, et al. A feasibility study evaluating rhBMP-2/absorbable collagen sponge for maxillary sinus floor augmentation. Int J Periodontics Restorative Dent 17:11-25, 1997.
26. Summary of Safety And Effectiveness Data, PMA P000058. Food and Drug Administration website: *http://www.fda.gov/cdrh/pdf/P000058b.pdf,* p 20. Posted July 11, 2002.
27. Burkus JK, Dorchak JD, Sanders DL. Radiographic assessment of interbody fusion using recombinant human bone morphogenetic protein type 2. Spine 28:372-377, 2003.

CHAPTER 5

Preclinical Efficacy of rhBMP-2 and ACS

Dosage and Concentration Selection

Questions about what volume, concentration, and dose of rhBMP-2 to use often occur. The volume of rhBMP-2/ACS required in a given bone grafting application should be of the same volume as autograft that would be required for that particular application. Therefore, a one-to-one relationship of rhBMP-2/ACS volume to autograft volume exists and is easy to remember. When surgically implanting the rhBMP-2/ACS, it is important to adequately fill the space in which new bone is desired, but not to overpack the sponge. Overpacking can result in hyperconcentration of the rhBMP-2 beyond what has been studied clinically.

Following the instructions for preparation in the rhBMP-2/ACS commercial kit results in a rhBMP-2 solution concentration of 1.5 mg/cc. This rhBMP-2 solution is evenly dispersed over a specific collagen sponge volume at the time of surgery. Consequently, dose or quantity of rhBMP-2 used surgically in a given bone grafting application is simply determined by multiplying the 1.5 mg/cc concentration of rhBMP-2 solution by the volume of collagen sponge carrier being used to fill the defect (Fig. 5-1). An example of this calculation is illustrated in Fig. 5-2, in which an interbody fusion cage, with an internal volume of 4 cc, is filled with 4 cc of collagen sponge saturated with 4 cc of the 1.5 mg/cc rhBMP-2 solution. This results in a total rhBMP-2 dose of 6 mg per cage.

Simply reporting the milligrams (mg) of BMP or the milligrams of BMP per gram of carrier (mg/g) when comparing results of different studies can be confusing and misleading. The reader is left uncertain as to whether the specified milligrams per gram of carrier are filling a 1 cc defect or a 20 cc defect. For this reason, all rhBMP-2 studies have reported the rhBMP-2 dosage in terms of milligrams per cubic centimeter (mg/cc).

Figure 5-1

Accurate determination of the rhBMP-2 dose is assessed based on a defined quantity of BMP contained in a defined volume.

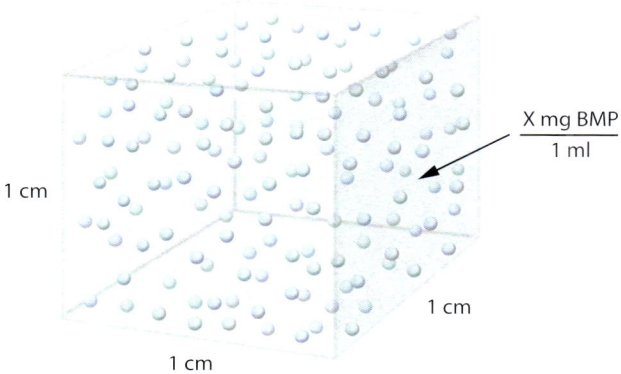

 Figure 5-2

Determination of rhBMP-2 delivered in a carrier. The carrier volume and the concentration of rhBMP-2 determine how much BMP is delivered in an interbody fusion technique.

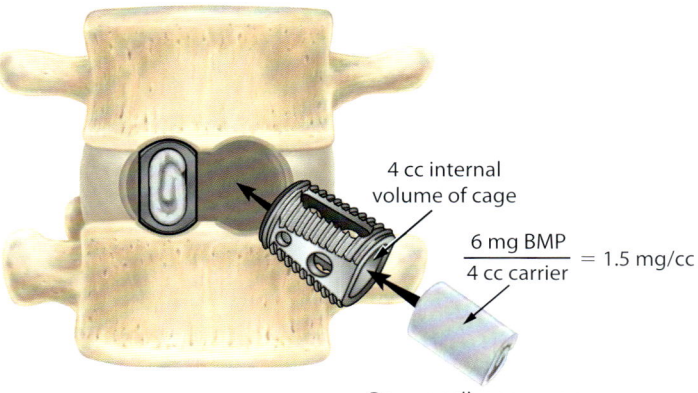

Species-Specific BMP Healing Rates

It was determined over years of research that the concentration of BMP required to produce the desired effect of new bone formation was species-dependent. The higher the species, the greater the concentrations of BMP required. The same dose that resulted in effective bone formation in a rat (0.05 mg/cc rhBMP-2/ACS) was found to be ineffective in monkeys. This suggests that the required BMP concentration is dependent on the species' bone formation and remodeling rate. For example, a rat will form bone in just 2 weeks with a concentration of only 0.05 mg/cc, whereas in monkeys approximately 1.0 mg/cc and 12 weeks are required to form bone (Table 5-1).

No data are yet available indicating whether the effective BMP concentration is specific to the anatomic location considered. For example, for a given species of animal, the same or very similar BMP concentrations have been used in both spinal fusion models and long bone fracture models, indicating that there may not be a concentration difference for effective

Table 5-1

BMP Concentrations Required for Different Species

Species	BMP Concentration (mg/cc)	Time to Fusion (wk)
Rat	0.01-0.05	2
Rabbit/dog	0.20-0.40	4-8
Monkey	0.6-0.8	12-24
Human	1.5-2.00	16-36

fusion for various bones in a given species. As more clinical experience is obtained with BMP, it is possible that more challenging anatomic surgical applications could require higher concentrations of BMP. For instance, the relatively short distance between the endplates of two vertebral bodies in an interbody spinal fusion is very different from the relatively large gap between two transverse processes in a posterolateral spinal fusion. In addition, the biologic environment of an interbody fusion is different from a posterolateral fusion. In the disc space, bleeding endplates provide a good source of osteogenic progenitor cells. In a posterolateral gutter, the decorticated surfaces of the transverse processes offer only a minimal area of bleeding bone, and the graft is surrounded by soft muscle tissue (Fig. 5-3).

Figure 5-3

Posterolateral fusion challenges. A posterolateral application offers the challenges of a larger gap to be fused and a minimal area of bleeding bone compared with an interbody fusion.

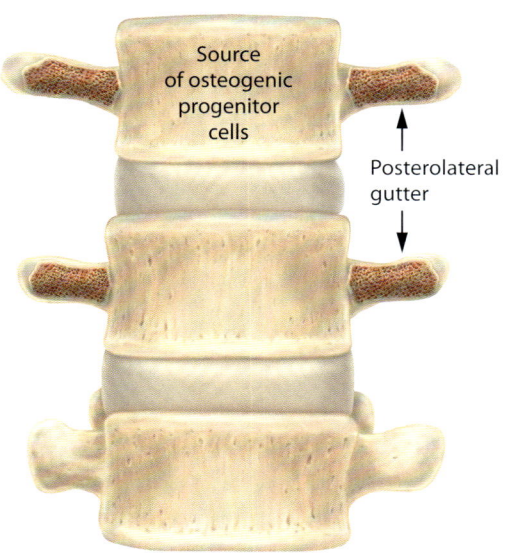

Other examples of more challenging clinical applications in which a higher concentration of BMP may be required include use in smokers and patients undergoing revision surgeries.

Techniques for Evaluating Spinal Fusions

It is important to be able to accurately evaluate the quality and quantity of spinal fusion masses when comparing different technologies for spinal fusion. Histologic studies allow investigators to directly assess the type and quantity of bone formation. However, histology is not available in human clinical studies. There is also an ongoing debate about using plain radiographs alone as a fusion assessment tool. Preclinical studies allow the unique ability to compare histologic and different methods of radiographic evaluation of the resulting fusion mass.

In a sheep study by Sandhu et al,[1] plain radiographs were demonstrated to be less effective at determining the amount of new bone formation compared with histology slides. The histologic results for the autograft control group determined that there was only a 37% fusion rate, while the plain radiographic results for the same group showed a 100% fusion rate. However, in the rhBMP-2/ACS group, plain radiographic and histologic evaluations both agreed that the fusion rate was 100%. Therefore, although plain radiographic and histologic results agreed for the rhBMP-2/ACS group, there was a wide gap between the two methods for the autograft group.

In the same sheep spinal fusion study, there was new bone growth in the animals implanted with rhBMP-2/ACS, rather than the formation of intervening soft tissue, which was the preponderant component in the autograft control animals. In this model, the rhBMP-2/ACS fusion mass had superior quality to the autograft fusion mass, when viewed histologically. The histologic method allowed for a better assessment of the bone quality, whereas plain radiographic assessment qualified both new bone and soft tissue as fusion masses.

Thin-slice CT scan technology is now available for assessing fusion success. Boden et al[2] compared thin-slice CT scans with histology for the ability to assess the quality of the fusion mass. In this study, using a rhesus monkey model, there was a strong correlation between the histology and the CT scans. It can therefore be concluded that thin-slice CT scans would provide a better assessment tool for determining fusion in clinical studies, compared with plain radiographs alone.

Preclinical rhBMP-2/ACS Interbody Studies With Metal Cages and Allograft Bone Dowels

The ultimate goal of interbody spinal fusion is to achieve bony fusion across a disc space that has been distracted to its normal height from a diseased, compressed state. At this time, there are no BMP carriers that can both sustain the loads for disc distraction and degrade or remodel as fusion occurs. Therefore, in the development of rhBMP-2 for interbody spinal fusion applications, research was conducted with the use of interbody constructs such as metallic cages or allograft bone dowels. These interbody constructs possess internal spaces normally packed with autologous bone graft to achieve a fusion across the disc space. The bone grafting material placed inside such interbody devices is not subjected to any significant loads or forces, eliminating the requirement that the carrier for BMP be load-bearing or resistant to minimal compressive forces.

Because there is one less design requirement for the carrier for interbody applications than for posterolateral fusion applications, development of rhBMP-2 for interbody spinal fusion was one of the first applications pursued clinically.

The carrier for rhBMP-2 used in the interbody fusion studies was a type I bovine absorbable collagen sponge (ACS). This cohesive sponge is hydrated with rhBMP-2 solution at the time of surgery. The rhBMP-2 binds to the collagen sponge, which is rolled up and placed into the interbody device cavity (Fig. 5-4).

The first preclinical interbody cage study using rhBMP-2 was reported by Sandhu et al.[1] This study compared the use of a single cylindrical cage filled with autograft from the iliac crest or rhBMP-2 on a collagen sponge carrier in the lumbar spine of sheep. The animals were sacrificed at 6 months. Fusion status was evaluated via radiographic and histologic analysis. Additionally, the explanted spines were biomechanically tested for fusion stiffness. The most definitive assessment of fusion was made

Figure 5-4

*Hydration and placement of the collagen sponge. **A**, The sponge is hydrated with the reconstituted rhBMP-2 solution. **B**, The hydrated sponge is rolled up and inserted into the cage.*

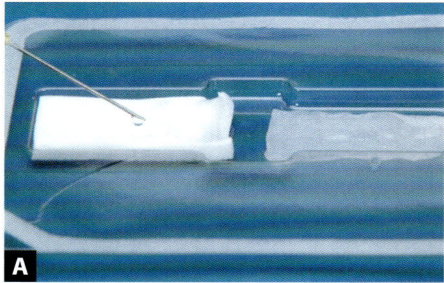
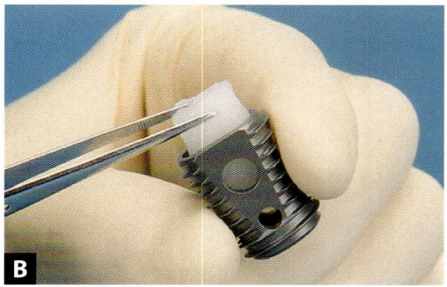

by the histologic findings, which revealed only a 37% fusion rate for autograft compared with 100% for rhBMP-2/ACS. The quality of the fusion was also better with rhBMP-2/ACS. Significantly less fibrous tissue was present in and around the cages than in cages filled with autograft (Fig. 5-5). In contrast, the plain radiographs of all cages in both groups appeared to indicate that fusion had occurred. As is becoming clinically evident, it is difficult to assess fusion status using plain radiographs, and this study confirmed that radiographs can overestimate the presence of fusion.

Figure 5-5

*rhBMP-2/ACS application results in a better quality of fusion. Histologic evaluation demonstrates the better fusion in the rhBMP-2 treatments (**A** and **B**) compared with the autograft control (**C** and **D**). Blue is bone tissue and pink is indicative of fibrous tissue.*

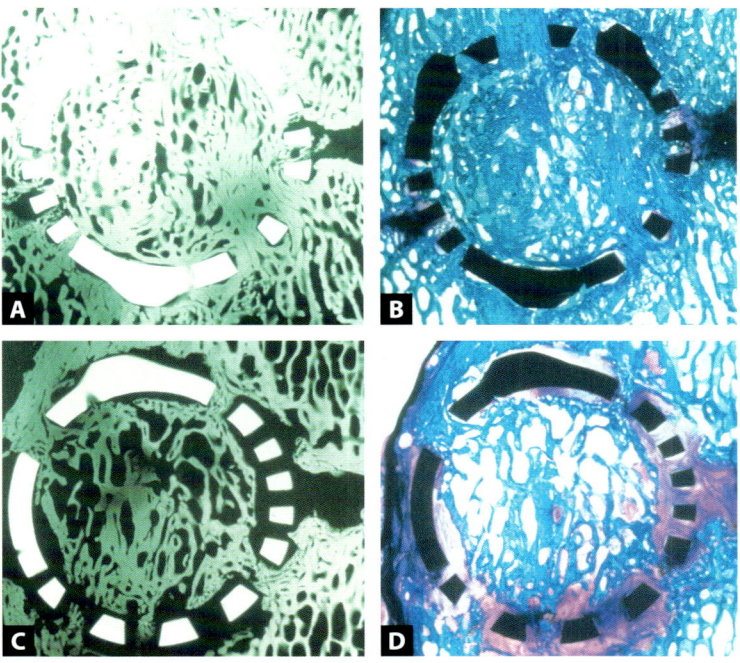

Figure 5-6

Radiographic evaluation compared with histologic evaluation of bone grafts in a goat model. Radiographic evaluations appear to overestimate the fusion results compared with the histologic evaluation. **A,** *Interbody fusion study in sheep: histologic findings showed 37% fusion for autograft compared with 100% fusion for rhBMP-2/ACS.* **B,** *Second fusion study in goats found 48% fusion in the autograft group and 95% in the rhBMP-2/ACS group.*

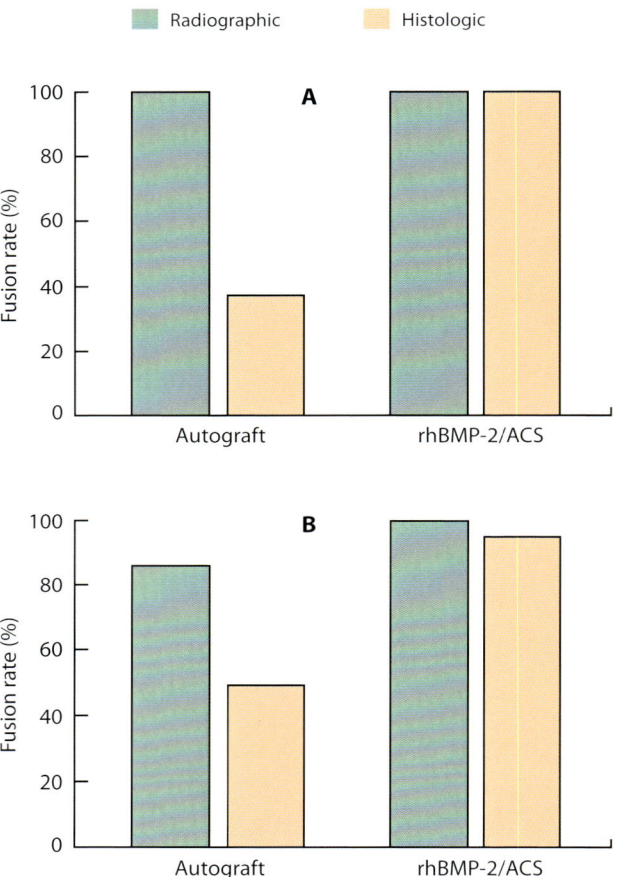

Numerous other preclinical interbody fusion studies using cages and rhBMP-2/ACS were subsequently conducted by other investigators and with similar findings. Zdeblick et al[3] conducted an interbody study with a titanium fusion cage in a goat model. The study compared autograft to rhBMP-2 delivered on a collagen sponge. The histologic fusion rates were very similar to those reported by Sandhu et al[1]: 48% for autograft and 95% for rhBMP-2. The investigators also noted that the radiographic evaluation of fusion status through a metal cage did not correlate to the histologic assessment of fusion (Fig. 5-6).

It was clear from the preclinical studies mentioned above that rhBMP-2/ACS was superior to autologous bone in interbody fusions with titanium cages.

Additional preclinical work was conducted using allograft bone dowels as the interbody construct instead of metal cages. Hecht et al[4] conducted a nonhuman primate study in which the use of rhBMP-2 with the collagen sponge carrier placed within allograft bone dowels was evaluated. The study treatment involved single-level interbody fusion with an allograft bone dowel with a central through-hole for packing bone graft. Three monkeys received iliac crest bone graft placed into the allograft bone dowel, and three others received rhBMP-2 on a collagen sponge. The duration of the study was 6 months. Fusion occurred in only one of the autograft control animals (33%). All rhBMP-2–treated animals had solid fusions. One interesting observation from this study was that by 6 months there had been complete remodeling and incorporation of the allograft into host bone in the rhBMP-2–treated animals (Fig. 5-7).

Before initiation of a human clinical trial with rhBMP-2 on the collagen sponge in a titanium lumbar interbody fusion cage, a nonhuman primate study was conducted by Boden et al[2] to select the rhBMP-2 concentration to be examined in the trial. Concentrations of 0, 0.75, and 1.50 mg/cc rhBMP-2 were tested in adult rhesus monkeys. At 6 months, none of the

Figure 5-7

*Allograft bone dowels filled with autograft compared with rhBMP-2/ACS-filled bone dowels. Histologic results reveal complete remodeling and incorporation of the allograft when rhBMP-2/ACS was used (**A** and **B**) compared with lack of fusion and incorporation in two thirds of the animals (monkeys) when iliac crest autograft was used (**C** and **D**).*

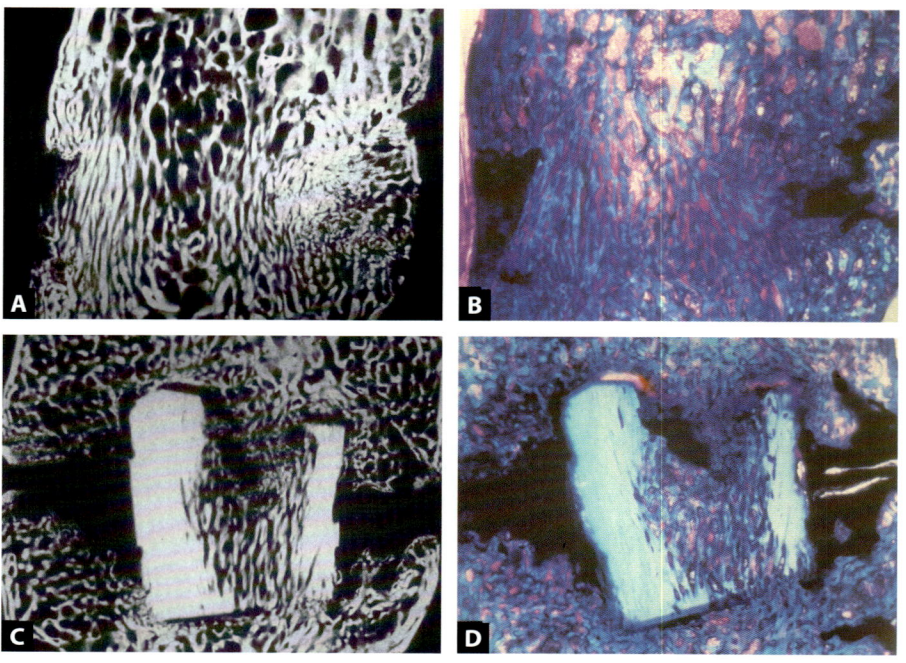

monkeys without the rhBMP-2 had evidence of fusion, compared with 100% of the monkeys given the rhBMP-2. The higher 1.50 mg/cc concentration appeared to result in slightly faster and denser bone formation than the lower 0.75 mg/cc concentration, without producing any adverse effects. Based on these results, 1.50 mg/cc was selected as the concentration to be used in the human clinical trial. The higher concentration accounted for the possible need for an increase in concentration when moving from use in rhesus monkeys to humans, similar to the increase in concentration needed when going from any lower species to a higher one. Table 5-2 lists some preclinical studies of rhBMP-2/ACS in interbody cages and allograft bone dowels.

Table 5-2

Summary of Interbody Fusion Preclinical Studies With rhBMP-2/ACS

Investigator	Species	Number of Subjects	Follow-up	Fusion Rate*
Sandhu et al[1]	Sheep	6-8/group	6 months	37% autograft 100% rhBMP-2/ACS
Zdeblick et al[3]	Goats	7/group	3 months	48% autograft 95% rhBMP-2/ACS
Hecht et al[4]	Monkeys	3/group	6 months	33% autograft 100% rhBMP-2/ACS
Boden et al[2]	Monkeys	3/group	6 months	0% sponge only 100% rhBMP-2/ACS

*Fusion assessed histologically in animal studies.

Comparisons With Iliac Crest Autograft: Rate and Quality of Fusion

The preclinical studies described in the previous section obtained results for rhBMP-2/ACS of 100% fusion in three studies and 95% fusion in one study. However, the autograft controls had fusion results varying from 37% to 48% in sheep and goats to 33% in the rhesus monkey, a higher-order species. One advantage of animal studies is the ability to assess the fusion rate and quality histologically. The sheep study by Sandhu et al[1] also discussed the quality of fusion obtained with rhBMP-2/ACS compared with autograft. The authors' assessment was that not only was the rate of fusion with rhBMP-2/ACS higher, but also the quality was judged to be superior. There was significantly less fibrous tissue present in and around the cages compared with the tissue in and around the autograft-filled cages. In the Hecht et al[4] study, the allograft bone dowel had been completely remodeled and incorporated into host bone when rhBMP-2/ACS was used to fill the allograft cavity.

In animal studies, the ability to assess bone quality through histology allows the conclusion that rhBMP-2/ACS produces higher quality bone than the bone produced when using autograft alone. The fusion and remodeling rates observed in the rhesus monkey model should be very similar to that in humans.

Recently, the quality and viability of autologous iliac crest bone grafts for spinal fusion have come into question. A large series of clinically failed interbody vertebral cages retrieved from humans were evaluated histologically.[5] In 78 cages retrieved from 48 patients, analysis revealed that the average area occupied by viable bone was only 44% (range, 0% to 80%).

The cages had been implanted for an average of 22 months. Fibrocartilage occupied up to 50% of the available area of the cages. Large pieces of cortical autograft were associated with only minimal new bone formation, whereas pieces of cancellous bone were associated with good formation. Although the scope of this study was limited to clinical failures, the research did illustrate the importance of autograft preparation as it relates to potential bone graft incorporation during spinal fusion.

Limitations of the Compressible Collagen Sponge Carrier

The application of rhBMP-2 for posterolateral fusions presents more challenges than does its use in interbody spinal fusion cages, which has resulted in a slightly longer developmental timeline. The carrier has an additional requirement to meet for posterolateral fusion: it must now resist compressive loads to preserve a three-dimensional physical space within the posterolateral gutter. Maintaining this space supports the formation of an adequate fusion mass/volume. The collagen sponge carrier performs well in cages, because it is not subjected to any compressive forces; however, when used in a posterolateral fusion application, it is subjected to compressive forces from the surrounding soft tissue, resulting in inadequate (or very thin) fusion mass/volume. Therefore specific bulking methods for using rhBMP-2 with the plain collagen sponge in posterolateral applications are being developed. At the same time, a search was undertaken for new compression-resistant carriers specifically designed for this application. INFUSE® Bone Graft should not be used alone for posterolateral fusions because of its compressibility.

As described in the FDA Summary of Safety and Effectiveness Data,[6] many lower-order animal studies involving rabbits and dogs have demonstrated the preclinical efficacy of rhBMP-2 in posterolateral fusion applications.[7-16] Table 5-3 lists more details of some of the preclinical studies of rhBMP-2/ACS and rhBMP-2/BCP carriers in posterolateral models referenced in the FDA Summary.

Table 5-3

Summary of Posterolateral Fusion Preclinical Studies With rhBMP-2

Investigator	Species	Number of Subjects	Follow-up	Fusion Rate (%)* or Fusion Volume (cc)
Schimandle et al[7]	Rabbit	9-12/group	5 wk	42% autograft 100% rhBMP-2 + autograft 100% rhBMP-2/ACS + autograft 100% rhBMP-2/ACS
Boden et al[17]	Rabbit	16/group	10 wk	100% rhBMP-2/ACS
Holliger et al[18]	Rabbit	9-12/group	4 wk	3.3 ml autograft 4.2 ml rhBMP-2/carrier
Suh et al[14]	Rabbit	14/group	5 wk	100% rhBMP-2/CRM (5:95) 100% rhBMP-2/CRM (60:40)

*Fusion assessed histologically in animal studies. Results in animal models may not be indicative of clinical performance.
BCP = 60% HA and 40% TCP.
ACS, Absorbable collagen sponge; *CRM*, compression-resistant matrix.

Table 5-3 (cont'd)

Summary of Posterolateral Fusion Preclinical Studies With rhBMP-2

Investigator	Species	Number of Subjects	Follow-up	Fusion Rate (%)* or Fusion Volume (cc)
Sandhu et al[8]	Dog	6/group	3 mo	0% autograft 100% rhBMP-2/carrier
Sandhu et al[20]	Dog	2-6/group	3 mo	100% rhBMP-2/carrier
Sheehan et al[19]	Dog	4/group	3 mo	1.2 ml autograft 6.6 ml rhBMP-2/carrier + autograft
Sandhu et al[9]	Dog	9-11/group	3 mo	89% undecorticated with rhBMP-2/carrier 100% decorticated with rhBMP-2/carrier
Fischgrund et al[10]	Dog	3/group	6 mo	8.6 ml autograft 21.9 ml rhBMP-2 + autograft 14.1 ml rhBMP-2/ACS + autograft 21.9 ml rhBMP-2
Helm et al[11]	Dog	6-10/group	6 mo	52% autograft 100% rhBMP-2 + autograft
David et al[16]	Dog	3/group	3 mo	33% autograft 100% rhBMP-2/ACS
Boden et al[13]	Monkey	2-6/group	6 mo	0% autograft 100% rhBMP-2/BCP
Suh et al[14]	Monkey	2/group	6 mo	0% rhBMP-2 (1.0 mg/cc)/CRM (5:95) 100% rhBMP-2 (2.0 mg/cc)/CRM (5:95) 100% rhBMP-2 (2.0 mg/cc)/CRM (15:85)

In the first of these studies, Schimandle et al[7] reported a 100% fusion rate for rhBMP-2 in a 4-week validated rabbit posterolateral fusion model, whereas the autograft controls had a fusion rate of only 42%. Greater and more rapid bone formation, consolidation, and remodeling were shown both radiographically and histologically with the use of rhBMP-2/ACS compared with autologous bone graft (Fig. 5-8). Fusions achieved with rhBMP-2 were biomechanically stronger and stiffer than autograft fusions (Fig. 5-9).

Figure 5-8

*rhBMP-2 improves fusion in a rabbit posterolateral fusion. A rabbit posterolateral fusion model reveals greater and more rapid bone formation, consolidation, and remodeling both histologically and radiographically when rhBMP-2/ACS was used (**A**), compared with autograft (**B**).*

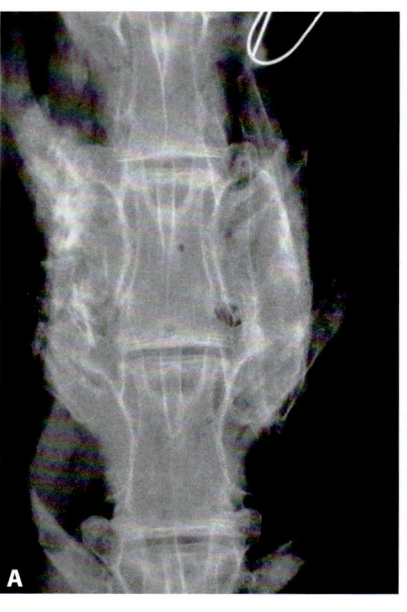
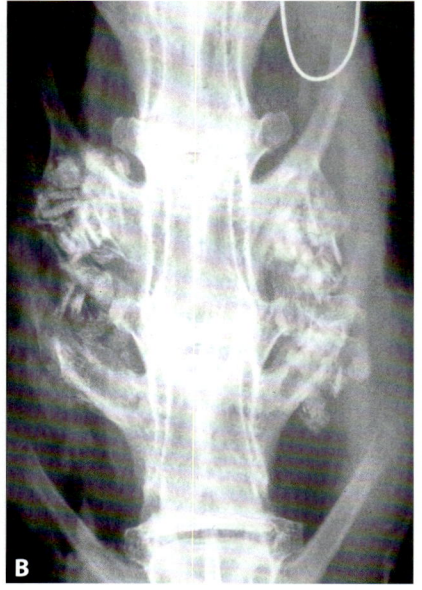

This work was soon followed by a study by Sandhu et al[8] reporting a 100% fusion rate in a 12-week canine posterolateral fusion model with the use of rhBMP-2; none of the autograft-treated control animals exhibited fusion. The investigators concluded that rhBMP-2 in this animal model is superior to autologous iliac crest bone in posterolateral fusions. The osteoinductive potency of rhBMP-2 was further demonstrated in a subsequent study conducted by Sandhu et al[9] using the same canine posterolateral fusion model without decortication. The investigators found no difference in fusion rate in undecorticated spines and decorticated spines treated with rhBMP-2. The higher rhBMP-2 doses evaluated resulted in 100% fusion rates with or without decortication in dogs. Results in animal models may not be indicative of clinical performance. Proper decortication and surgical technique should always be maintained when using INFUSE® Bone Graft.

Figure 5-9

Strength and stiffness were measured in a rabbit posterolateral fusion model. Autograft achieved significantly lower values in both strength and stiffness compared with rhBMP-2.

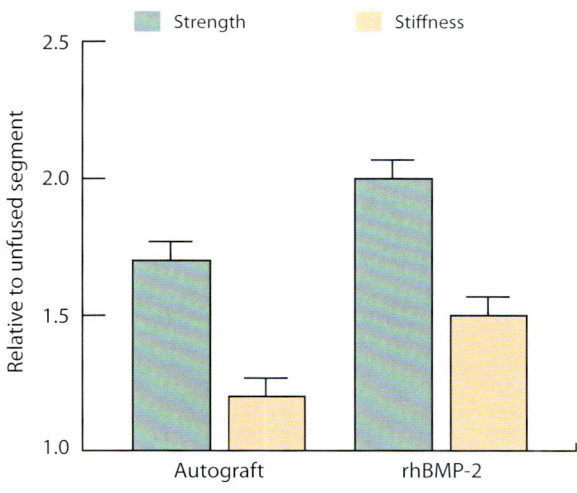

rhBMP-2 as a Possible Graft Enhancer

A few investigators have studied the potential to use rhBMP-2 as a supplement to autologous bone graft in posterolateral fusions. Fischgrund et al[10] evaluated in a canine model the use of rhBMP-2 either applied as a solution directly onto autologous bone graft or applied on a collagen sponge and subsequently mixed with autologous bone graft. These treatments were compared with autologous bone graft alone; final fusion mass volumes were compared based on quantitative CT analysis. Significantly larger fusion mass volumes resulted with the application of rhBMP-2 to the autologous bone graft; an even larger difference was seen in the group in which the rhBMP-2 solution was applied to the collagen sponge first (Fig. 5-10).

 Figure 5-10

Augmentation of autograft using rhBMP-2 in a canine spinal fusion model. Volumetric measurements of the total fusion mass (cubic centimeters) were determined by using CT scanning after 8 weeks. Autograft volume when used alone is compared with autograft with rhBMP-2.

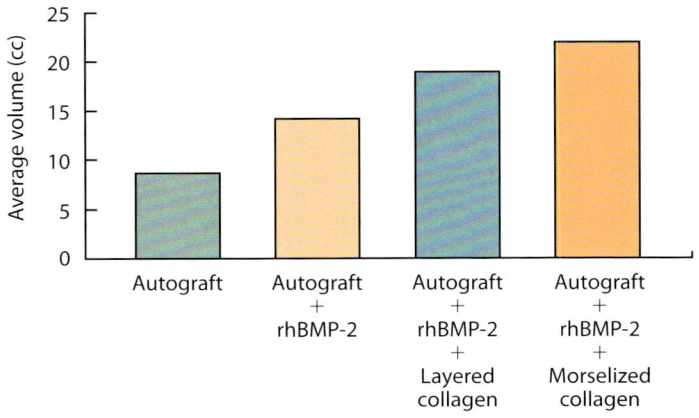

Helm et al[11] also compared autologous bone graft with autologous bone graft supplemented with rhBMP-2 in a canine model. CT films were used to measure the fusion mass volume and quantify changes from the initial postoperative volume. At 24 weeks postoperatively, the autologous bone graft fusion mass volume only increased 0.26 cc, whereas the rhBMP-2–supplemented autologous bone graft fusion mass volume increased 10.42 cc. This difference was statistically significant ($p = 0.036$) (Fig. 5-11).

Figure 5-11

Mass volume of bone deposition is considerably increased when autograft is supplemented with rhBMP-2.

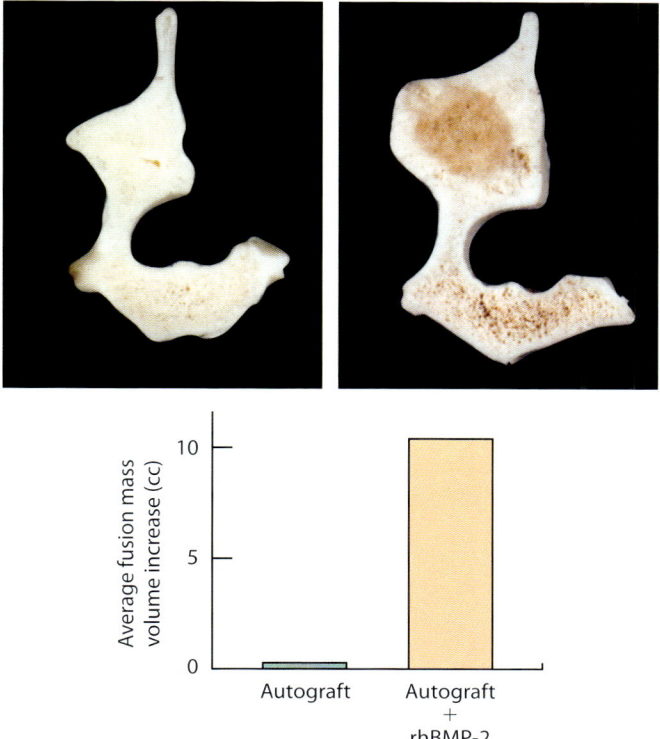

In all of these previously discussed posterolateral studies, the ACS carrier was the same material used in the interbody cage fusion studies. Recognizing that these preclinical efficacy studies were conducted in lower animals, the next step in evaluating rhBMP-2 for posterolateral fusions was to confirm the efficacy of rhBMP-2 on the plain collagen sponge carrier in a higher-order animal that has a slower bone formation rate that is closer to that of humans. A rhesus monkey study was conducted by Martin et al[12] with the collagen sponge carrier at various doses and concentrations to establish the parameters for ensuring the safety of the collagen sponge carrier in a posterolateral fusion application. It was found that rhBMP-2 concentrations and doses that were effective in lower animals (0.43 mg/cc and 2.0 mg, respectively), while safe, were not effective in posterolateral fusions in primates. Results of this study revealed that both the rhBMP-2 concentration and the delivered dose had to be increased to reliably achieve successful fusions. It was hypothesized that in higher-order animals in which the bone formation process is slower, the overlying paraspinal muscles compressed the collagen sponge before new bone formed within its porous matrix. The resulting bone mass was too thin to be considered a successful spinal fusion.

Preclinical rhBMP-2 Posterolateral Studies: Use of Bulking Agents

Boden et al[13] conducted a nonhuman primate posterolateral fusion study using biphasic calcium phosphate (BCP) ceramic blocks with rhBMP-2 in comparison with autograft. The porous BCP blocks, which had a composition of 60% hydroxyapatite (HA) and 40% tricalcium phosphate (TCP), were soaked directly in rhBMP-2. The rhBMP-2 concentrations on the BCP blocks tested were 0.0, 1.5, 2.0, and 3.0 mg/cc. At 6 months, fusion had occurred in all monkeys treated with rhBMP-2, but fusion had not occurred in any of the autograft-treated animals. Although the results of this nonhuman primate study were promising and showed preclinical efficacy, the slow resorption rate of the BCP blocks made it difficult to monitor the progression of fusion on radiographs. In addition, the brittle ceramic blocks were difficult to shape intraoperatively, leaving little room for error in positioning them.

Suh et al[14] evaluated the preclinical efficacy of a compression-resistant matrix (CRM) as a carrier for rhBMP-2. HA/TCP granules were combined with the ACS, and posterolateral fusion was assessed in both rabbits and non-human primates. The ceramic composition of the HA/TCP granules tested was at a ratio of either 15:85, 5:95, or 60:40. In addition, different rhBMP-2 concentrations were evaluated (1.0 or 2.0 mg/cc). After assessing the outcomes using radiographs, manual palpation, undecalcified histology, and biomechanical testing, the authors concluded that the 15:85 HA/TCP ratio demonstrated the preclinical efficacy of a rhBMP-2 concentration of 2.0 mg/cc. This study demonstrated the feasibility of rhBMP-2/CRM (2.0 mg/cc) in inducing posterolateral fusions in non-human primates. This rhBMP-2 formulation is currently under investigation in a prospective, randomized FDA-approved IDE clinical study in humans.

All of these preclinical posterolateral studies, are presented as supporting information relevant to the intended clinical use of rhBMP-2/ACS in lumbar interbody fusions with a cage.

 Effect on Spinal Tissue

The studies described in Chapters 3 and 4 provide information on the safety profile of rhBMP-2 and rhBMP-2/ACS, but they do not address concerns that may be specific to the use of rhBMP-2 in spinal applications. Therefore, a study was initiated to assess the effects of rhBMP-2/ACS on exposed dura and neural tissue after standard decompressive lumbar laminectomy using a canine model.[15] This study represented a worst-case model in which the rhBMP-2/ACS is in direct contact with the spinal cord. Twenty skeletally mature beagles underwent a spinal laminectomy at the L4-5 level. Half of the animals also received a "dural nick" made with a 22-gauge needle in the posterior midline of the spinal cord until cerebrospinal fluid was noted to egress from the nick. Then either autologous bone graft or rhBMP-2/ACS was implanted directly on the exposed spinal cord in the laminectomy defect. Animals were randomized to one of four treatment groups:

1. Autologous morselized corticocancellous rib graft without dural nick (n = 5)
2. Autologous morselized corticocancellous rib graft with dural nick (n = 5)
3. 0.10 mg/cc rhBMP-2/ACS without dural nick (n = 5)
4. 0.10 mg/cc rhBMP-2/ACS with dural nick (n = 5)

Animals were sacrificed at 12 weeks. Evaluation consisted of clinical, neurologic, and radiographic examination and histologic analysis. The clinical examination involved weekly body weight monitoring, monthly blood tests, and cerebrospinal fluid analysis at necropsy. Neurologic assessment consisted of weekly observations of the animal's gait, placing reflex, patellar reflex, and pain withdrawal reflex of both hind limbs. Radiographs were taken on a monthly basis to assess changes in the spinal cord, surrounding spinal canal, and graft material using preestablished measurement parameters. Histologic studies were used to assess the effect of rhBMP-2/ACS in direct contact with neurologic tissue.

Neither rhBMP-2/ACS nor the dural nick caused deleterious results in these animals. The implants resulted in a physical depression of the dural membrane that was radiographically apparent, suggesting that the implant came to rest adjacent to the thecal sac. The rhBMP-2/ACS induced bone growth around the margin of the spinal canal, suggesting that the rhBMP-2 came in direct contact with the dural membrane and may even have leaked into the neuroforamen, because a bony reaction was noted there. There was no evidence of mineralization within the thecal sac and no clinical evidence of any neurologic abnormalities in these animals (Figs. 5-12 and 5-13). No evidence of any clinical abnormalities was noted in these animals based on blood and cerebrospinal fluid analyses.

David et al[16] evaluated the potential of spinal canal or nerve root encroachment in rhBMP-2/ACS–treated dogs and found no evidence of any encroachment in the rhBMP-2 groups. All rhBMP-2/ACS groups had better fusions at 3 months than the autogenous bone group. In addition, no ectopic bone formation was found in any paravertebral soft tissue. A rhesus monkey study (Hecht et al[4]) also demonstrated that the foraminal spaces and nerves were maintained in the rhBMP-2/ACS–treated group. There was no foraminal encroachment by the *de novo* bone formation. In addition, no spinal canal stenosis was evidenced in the medial sections. This result was maintained at the 6-month time period. Moreover, there were no inflammatory or immune responses evidenced in the histology of the rhBMP-2/ACS group, in contrast with the autograft control group.

The results from primate studies are more indicative of human results, as bone formation and remodeling rates in humans are much closer to those of the rhesus monkey than those of dogs. Martin et al[12] reported that the presence of a laminectomy defect with exposed dura did not preclude the safe use of rhBMP-2. The study also confirmed that the carrier is of

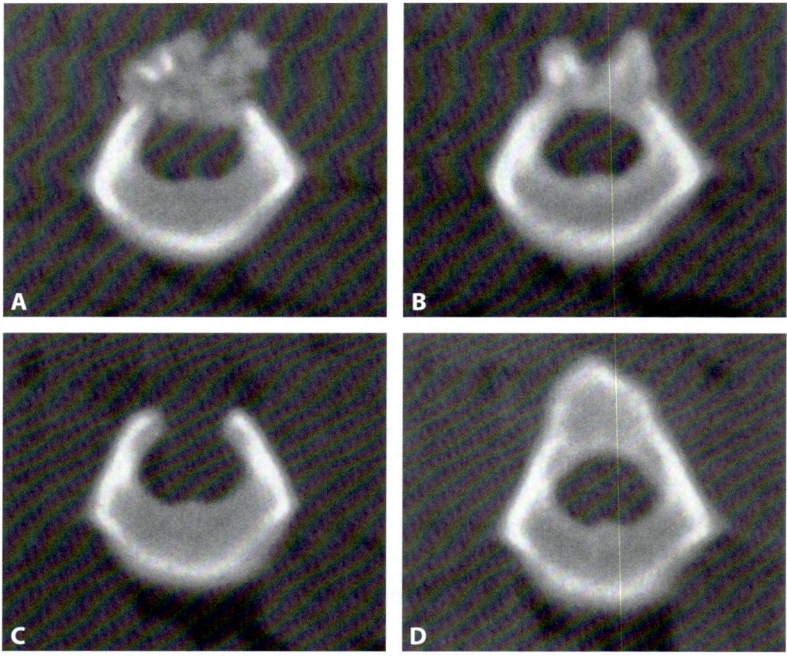

Figure 5-12

*CT images at the level of the laminectomy in dogs. **A**, Dog treated with autograft bone has evidence of bone fragments immediately after surgery. **B**, Fragments coalesced into a single bone mass at 3 months. **C**, The rhBMP-2/ACS implant does not image immediately after surgery. **D**, A mineralized mass can be seen at 3 months. There was no CT evidence of bone forming within the dura or in the spinal cord.*

paramount importance to retain the rhBMP-2, because less optimal carriers resulted in bone formation outside the target area. When using rhBMP-2 with the ACS sponge, the use did not lead to bone overgrowth in the spinal canal; neither did it preclude performing a laminectomy.

Figure 5-13

Histologic views of the lamina and spinal canal 3 months after surgery. *A,* Photomicrographs of an rhBMP-2/ACS implanted dog. *B,* Photomicrographs of an autograft-implanted animal.

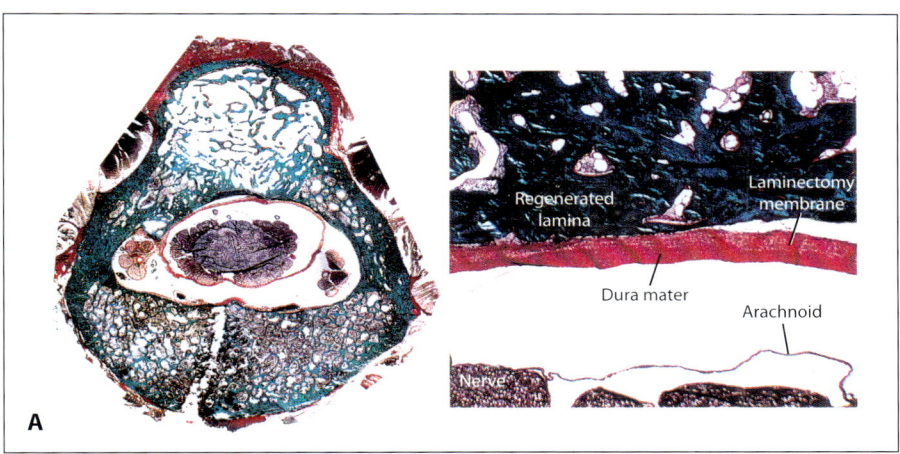
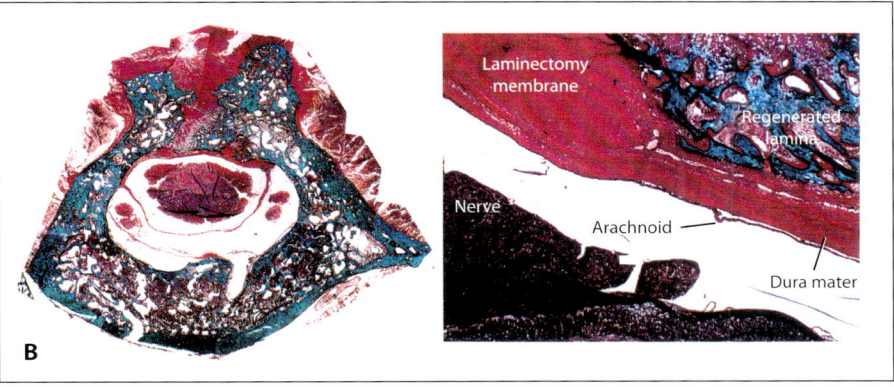

Frequently Asked Questions

What are the risks associated with implanting a genetically engineered biologic protein? Has the presence of rhBMP-2 in the body led to any implant, systemic, or reproductive toxicity?

The half-life of rhBMP-2 in the human blood stream is only seconds, and it is excreted from the body via the urine. To date, there is no evidence that the presence of rhBMP-2 causes any form of toxicity in the body.

Will a larger dosage of INFUSE® Bone Graft give more fusion?

Animal studies indicate that no further benefit is achieved after the threshold level has been achieved.

What data exist for effects on the dura?

Several animal studies have examined the dura and neural cord after deliberate exposure to rhBMP-2 without seeing negative effects (see Figs. 5-12 and 5-13).

Could there be unwanted bone growth away from intended site?

It has been demonstrated that rhBMP-2 does not have systemic activity. Additionally, in contrast to findings in the animal studies, it has been demonstrated that bleeding bone is necessary for human bone osteogenesis. The combination of rhBMP-2 and the bleeding bone initiates new bone formation.

In clinical studies, no ectopic bone formation occurred that was not directly adjacent to the surgical site. No clinical complications due to ectopic bone formation have occurred. No ectopic bone formation occurred in the ALIF study. Moreover, no bone formed remote from the surgical site in any patient receiving rhBMP-2 with ACS.

The safety and effectiveness of the INFUSE® Bone Graft component with other spinal implants, implanted at locations other than the lower lumbar spine or used in surgical techniques other than the anterior open approach (LT-CAGE®, INTER FIX®, INTER FIX™ RP Devices) have not been established.

- When degenerative disc disease was treated by a posterior lumbar interbody fusion procedures with stand-alone cylindrical threaded cages (INTER FIX™ devices), posterior bone formation was observed in some instances.

REFERENCES

1. Sandhu HS, Kabo JM, Turner AS, et al. rhBMP-2 augmentation of titanium fusion cages for experimental anterior lumbar fusion. Presented at the Eleventh Annual Meeting of the North American Spine Society, Vancouver, BC, Oct 1996.
2. Boden SD, Martin GJ Jr, Horton WC, et al. Laparoscopic anterior spinal arthrodesis with rhBMP-2 in a titanium interbody threaded cage. J Spinal Disord 11:95-101, 1998.
3. Zdeblick TA, Ghanayem AJ, Rapoff AJ, et al. Cervical interbody fusion cages. An animal model with and without bone morphogenetic protein. Spine 23:758-765; discussion 766, 1998.
4. Hecht BP, Fischgrund JS, Herkowitz HN, et al. The use of recombinant human bone morphogenetic protein 2 (rhBMP-2) to promote spinal fusion in a nonhuman primate anterior interbody fusion model. Spine 24:629-636, 1999.
5. Togawa D, Bauer TW, Lieberman IH, et al. Lumbar intervertebral body fusion cages: Histological evaluation of clinically failed cages retrieved from humans. J Bone Joint Surg Am 86:70-79, 2004.
6. FDA Summary of Safety and Effectiveness Data, INFUSE® Bone Graft/LT-CAGE® Lumbar Tapered Fusion Device, July 2, 2002, P000058.
7. Schimandle JH, Boden SD, Hutton WC. Experimental spinal fusion with recombinant human bone morphogenetic protein-2. Spine 20:1326-1337, 1995.
8. Sandhu HS, Kanim LE, Kabo JM, et al. Evaluation of rhBMP-2 with an OPLA carrier in a canine posterolateral (transverse process) spinal fusion model. Spine 20:2669-2682, 1995.
9. Sandhu HS, Kanim LE, Toth JM, et al. Experimental spinal fusion with recombinant human bone morphogenetic protein-2 without decortication of osseous elements. Spine 22:1171-1180, 1997. Erratum in Spine 22:2463, 1997.

10. Fischgrund JS, James SB, Chabot MC, et al. Augmentation of autograft using rhBMP-2 and different carrier media in the canine spinal fusion model. J Spinal Disord 10:467-472, 1997.
11. Helm GA, Sheehan JM, Sheehan JP, et al. Utilization of type I collagen gel, demineralized bone matrix, and bone morphogenetic protein-2 to enhance autologous bone lumbar spinal fusion. J Neurosurg 86:93-100, 1997.
12. Martin GJ Jr, Boden SD, Morone MA, et al. Posterolateral intertransverse process spinal arthrodesis with rhBMP-2 in a nonhuman primate: Important lessons learned regarding dose, carrier, and safety. J Spinal Disord 12:179-186, 1999.
13. Boden SD, Martin GJ Jr, Morone MA, et al. Posterolateral lumbar intertransverse process spine arthrodesis with recombinant human bone morphogenetic protein 2/hydroxyapatite-tricalcium phosphate after laminectomy in the nonhuman primate. Spine 24:1179-1185, 1999.
14. Suh DY, Boden SD, Louis-Ugbo J, et al. Delivery of recombinant human bone morphogenetic protein-2 using a compression-resistant matrix in posterolateral spine fusion in the rabbit and in the non-human primate. Spine 27:353-360, 2002.
15. Meyer RA Jr, Gruber HE, Howard BA, et al. Safety of recombinant human bone morphogenetic protein-2 after spinal laminectomy in the dog. Spine 24:747-754, 1999.
16. David SM, Gruber HE, Meyer RA Jr, et al. Lumbar spinal fusion using recombinant human bone morphogenetic protein in the canine. A comparison of three dosages and two carriers. Spine 24:1973-1979, 1999.
17. Boden SD, Moskovitz PA, Morone MA, et al. Video-assisted lateral intertransverse process arthrodesis. Validation of a new minimally invasive lumbar spinal fusion technique in the rabbit and nonhuman primate (rhesus) models. Spine 21:2689-2697, 1996.
18. Holliger EH, Trawick RH, Boden SD, et al. Morphology of the lumbar intertransverse process fusion mass in the rabbit model: A comparison between two bone graft materials—rhBMP-2 and autograft. J Spinal Disord 9:125-128, 1996.
19. Sheehan JP, Kallmes DF, Sheehan JM, et al. Molecular methods of enhancing lumbar spine fusion. Neurosurgery 39:548-554, 1996.
20. Sandhu HS, Kanim LE, Kabo JM, et al. Effective doses of recombinant human bone morphogenetic protein-2 in experimental spinal fusion. Spine 21:2115-2122, 1996.

CHAPTER 6

Clinical Efficacy of rhBMP-2/ACS

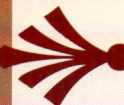

The previous chapters reviewed and described the technology, safety, and preclinical data for rhBMP-2 and rhBMP-2/ACS used in spinal fusion. The animal spinal fusion studies lent confidence to the design of clinical studies necessary to gain FDA approval for the use of this biotechnology in humans. Taking the studies step-by-step from lower animals to non-human primates provided a firm foundation for and clarified the goals and expectations of clinical studies. The clinical studies are therefore the culminating step in a long and arduous process of cultivating a promising technology all the way to a realized medical solution, but a step that could not have been safely taken without the preceding studies. The clinical studies ultimately led to FDA approval of INFUSE® Bone Graft/LT-CAGE® Lumbar Tapered Fusion Device on July 2, 2002 (PMA Number P000058) (Medtronic Sofamor Danek, Memphis, TN). That approval was supplemented in December 2003 to also include certain INTER FIX™ Threaded Fusion Devices. The Brief Summary of Indications, Contraindications, and Warnings for the INFUSE® Bone Graft/Interbody Fusion Device is shown in Fig. 6-1.

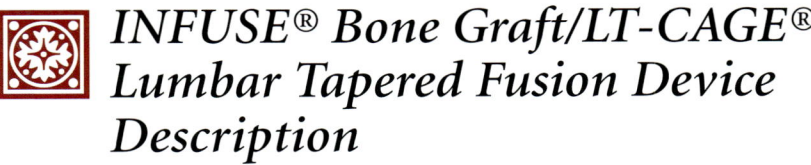 INFUSE® Bone Graft/LT-CAGE® Lumbar Tapered Fusion Device Description

The INFUSE® Bone Graft/LT-CAGE® Lumbar Tapered Fusion Device consists of a tapered metallic spinal fusion cage, rhBMP-2, and an ACS carrier/scaffold to which the rhBMP-2 is applied at the time of surgery. The INFUSE® Bone Graft component is inserted into the LT-CAGE® Lumbar Tapered Fusion Device component to form the complete INFUSE® Bone Graft/LT-CAGE® Lumbar Tapered Fusion Device. These components must be used as a system (Fig. 6-2).

Figure 6-1

Brief summary of indications, contraindications, and warnings for the INFUSE® Bone Graft/Interbody Fusion Device.

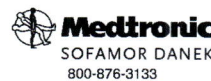

 Figure 6-2

The INFUSE® Bone Graft/LT-CAGE® Lumbar Tapered Fusion Device.

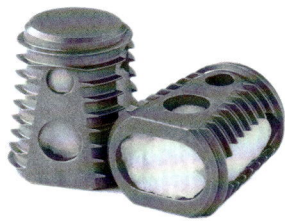

The LT-CAGE® Device consists of a hollow, perforated, machined cylinder with opposing flat sides. The cage has a tapered design with an angle of 8.8 degrees and is available in diameters ranging from 14 to 18 mm at the narrow end of the taper and 17 to 22 mm at the wide end of the taper. It is available in lengths ranging from 20 to 26 mm. There are two holes on each of the two flat sides. On each of the two rounded aspects, there is a single rounded slot. The implants have a helical screw thread on the outer surface. One end of the device is closed. The other end is open to be filled with the INFUSE® Bone Graft component. The LT-CAGE® implants are made from implant grade titanium alloy (Ti-6Al-4V).

INFUSE® Bone Graft consists of recombinant human bone morphogenetic protein-2 (rhBMP-2, also known as dibotermin alfa) placed on an absorbable collagen sponge (ACS). The INFUSE® Bone Graft component induces new bone tissue formation at the site of implantation. The active agent in the INFUSE® Bone Graft component is the rhBMP-2.

The ACS is a soft, white, pliable, and absorbent implantable matrix. The ACS is made from bovine type I collagen obtained from the deep flexor (Achilles) tendons of steers. The ACS acts as a carrier for the rhBMP-2 and as a scaffold for new bone formation.

Three volume sizes of the INFUSE® Bone Graft component are available based on the internal volume of the fusion device component that is selected (Fig. 6-3). Each kit contains all the components necessary to prepare the INFUSE® Bone Graft component: the rhBMP-2 (which must be reconstituted), sterile water, absorbable collagen sponge(s), syringes with needles, the package insert, and instructions for preparation. The number of each item may vary depending on the size of the kit. Note that the Large II kit configuration is also sold in Europe under the trade name InductOs™ (Wyeth Europa Ltd, United Kingdom) and has specific indications related to its European approval (available through local Medtronic offices).

The rhBMP-2 is provided as a filter-sterilized, lyophilized powder in vials delivering either 4.2 mg or 12 mg of protein. After appropriate reconstitution, both configurations result in the same formulation and concentration (1.5 mg/cc) of rhBMP-2. The solution is then applied to the provided absorbable collagen sponge(s). The INFUSE® Bone Graft component is prepared at the time of surgery and allowed a prescribed amount of time to bind (no less than 15 minutes) before placement inside the LT-CAGE® Lumbar Tapered Fusion Device components.

INFUSE® Bone Graft/LT-CAGE® Lumbar Tapered Fusion Device Pilot Clinical Study Results

In 1997, Medtronic Sofamor Danek initiated a pilot human Investigational Device Exemption (IDE) clinical trial with rhBMP-2 on a collagen sponge (1.5 mg/cc rhBMP-2/ACS; INFUSE® Bone Graft) in the LT-CAGE® Lumbar Tapered Fusion Device using an anterior surgical approach. Anterior

Figure 6-3

The appropriate INFUSE® Bone Graft kit for the corresponding LT-CAGE® Lumbar Tapered Fusion Device component size.

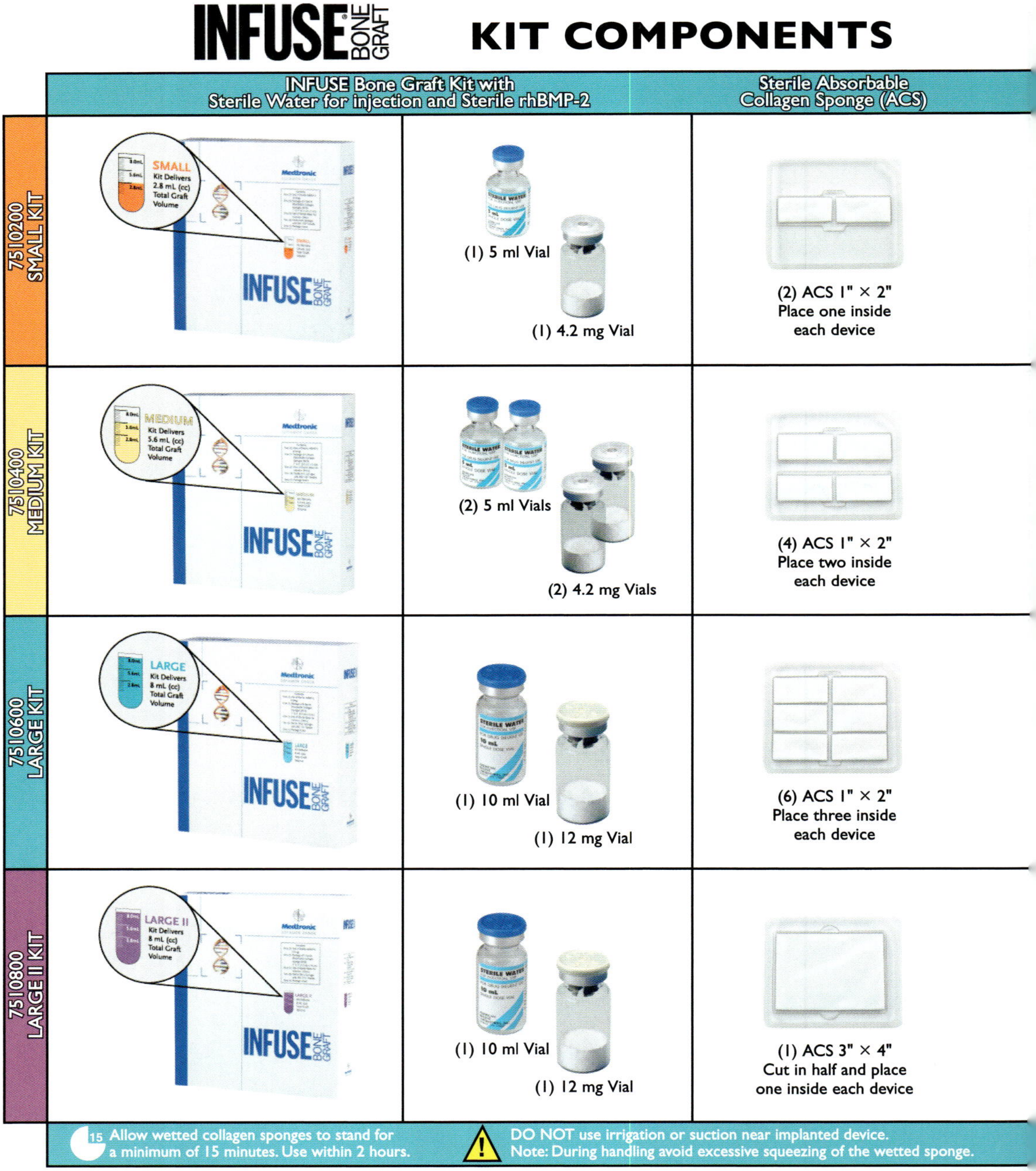

INFUSE® BONE GRAFT KIT COMPONENTS

Kit	INFUSE Bone Graft Kit with Sterile Water for injection and Sterile rhBMP-2	Sterile Absorbable Collagen Sponge (ACS)
7510200 SMALL KIT — SMALL Kit Delivers 2.8 mL (cc) Total Graft Volume	(1) 5 ml Vial; (1) 4.2 mg Vial	(2) ACS 1" × 2" Place one inside each device
7510400 MEDIUM KIT — MEDIUM Kit Delivers 5.6 mL (cc) Total Graft Volume	(2) 5 ml Vials; (2) 4.2 mg Vials	(4) ACS 1" × 2" Place two inside each device
7510600 LARGE KIT — LARGE Kit Delivers 8 mL (cc) Total Graft Volume	(1) 10 ml Vial; (1) 12 mg Vial	(6) ACS 1" × 2" Place three inside each device
7510800 LARGE II KIT — LARGE II Kit Delivers 8 mL (cc) Total Graft Volume	(1) 10 ml Vial; (1) 12 mg Vial	(1) ACS 3" × 4" Cut in half and place one inside each device

15 Allow wetted collagen sponges to stand for a minimum of 15 minutes. Use within 2 hours.

⚠ **DO NOT** use irrigation or suction near implanted device. Note: During handling avoid excessive squeezing of the wetted sponge.

AND GRAFT VOLUME GUIDE

Typical Vertebral Gap Measurements	LT-CAGE® Device	INTER FIX™ Device	INTER FIX™ RP Device	INTER FIX™ RP Device with INTER FIX™ Device
~12 mm to 16 mm Total Graft Volume 2.8 ml (cc)	14 mm × 20 mm 14 mm × 23 mm 16 mm × 20 mm	12 mm × 20 mm 12 mm × 25 mm 14 mm × 20 mm 14 mm × 23 mm 14 mm × 26 mm 14 mm × 29 mm 16 mm × 20 mm 16 mm × 23 mm	12 mm × 20 mm 12 mm × 25 mm 14 mm × 20 mm 14 mm × 23 mm 14 mm × 26 mm 14 mm × 29 mm 16 mm × 20 mm 16 mm × 23 mm	12 mm × 20 mm 12 mm × 25 mm 14 mm × 20 mm 14 mm × 23 mm 14 mm × 26 mm 14 mm × 29 mm 16 mm × 20 mm 16 mm × 23 mm
~16 mm to 20 mm Total Graft Volume 5.6 ml (cc)	16 mm × 23 mm 16 mm × 26 mm 18 mm × 23 mm	16 mm × 26 mm 16 mm × 29 mm 18 mm × 20 mm 18 mm × 23 mm 18 mm × 26 mm 18 mm × 29 mm 20 mm × 20 mm 20 mm × 23 mm	16 mm × 26 mm 16 mm × 29 mm 18 mm × 20 mm 18 mm × 23 mm 18 mm × 26 mm 18 mm × 29 mm 20 mm × 20 mm 20 mm × 23 mm 20 mm × 26 mm 20 mm × 29 mm 22 mm × 20 mm 22 mm × 23 mm	16 mm × 26 mm 16 mm × 29 mm 18 mm × 20 mm 18 mm × 23 mm 18 mm × 26 mm 18 mm × 29 mm 20 mm × 20 mm 20 mm × 23 mm
~20 mm to 24 mm Total Graft Volume 8.0 ml (cc)	18 mm × 26 mm	20 mm × 26 mm 20 mm × 29 mm 22 mm × 20 mm 22 mm × 23 mm 24 mm × 20 mm	22 mm × 26 mm 22 mm × 29 mm 24 mm × 20 mm 24 mm × 23 mm	20 mm × 26 mm 20 mm × 29 mm 22 mm × 20 mm 22 mm × 23 mm 22 mm × 26 mm 22 mm × 29 mm 24 mm × 20 mm 24 mm × 23 mm
~20 mm to 24 mm Total Graft Volume 8.0 ml (cc)	18 mm × 26 mm	20 mm × 26 mm 20 mm × 29 mm 22 mm × 20 mm 22 mm × 23 mm 24 mm × 20 mm	22 mm × 26 mm 22 mm × 29 mm 24 mm × 20 mm 24 mm × 23 mm	20 mm × 26 mm 20 mm × 29 mm 22 mm × 20 mm 22 mm × 23 mm 22 mm × 26 mm 22 mm × 29 mm 24 mm × 20 mm 24 mm × 23 mm

INFUSE® Bone Graft in combination with LT-CAGE®, INTER FIX™ or INTER FIX™ RP devices incorporate technology developed by Gary K. Michelson, MD.

lumbar interbody fusion (ALIF) is an effective surgical treatment of patients with symptomatic degenerative disc disease (DDD). Fusion of the degenerative and unstable segment can give significant relief from this disabling and often progressive condition. The anterior approach to the lumbosacral spine enables the surgeon to expand the disc space and re-establish the normal anatomic alignment. The FDA required a pilot IDE clinical trial to assess the safety of INFUSE® Bone Graft before initiating a large multicenter pivotal IDE clinical trial. The pilot study was a prospective, randomized clinical trial in which the investigational and control patients were enrolled 3:1. It consisted of 14 patients: 11 were treated with INFUSE® Bone Graft and three were treated with iliac crest autograft. Zdeblick et al[1] reported interim results and Boden et al[2] reported the 2-year results of this study.

Based on radiographic review by three independent radiologists, fusion occurred in all the patients treated with INFUSE® Bone Graft, whereas in one of the autograft-treated patients, fusion failed to occur. Assessment of fusion was made easier with the use of thin-slice CT reconstructions. Comparison of a given patient's CTs over time permitted determination of biologic activity inside the cages and whether it was progressing toward fusion. This was particularly true for the rhBMP-2–treated patients since the BMP-soaked sponge is initially radiolucent on implantation. Autograft-filled cages appear radiopaque immediately after the procedure; therefore changes within the cages over time are much more subtle and difficult to observe. Examples from this pilot of a patient treated with INFUSE® Bone Graft and a patient treated with autograft are shown in Fig. 6-4.

The general Oswestry Low Back Pain Disability Questionnaire (assessment scale 0 to 100) was used to assess clinical outcome. This is a well-accepted general pain assessment in which patients report the effect of their level of pain on the activities of daily living. According to the FDA-approved protocol, the Oswestry score had to be reduced by 15 points from the preoperative score for the patient's outcome to be considered a success. At 24 months, the autograft control patients had an Oswestry success rate of 66% (two of three), and the INFUSE® Bone Graft investigational patients had a 90.9% success rate (10 of 11). The mean improvement in Oswestry score for the INFUSE® Bone Graft patients was 25 points (71.8%) at 24 months, compared with a 15-point (54.1%) improvement in control patients.

The presence of antibodies to rhBMP-2 and bovine and human type I collagen was assessed. Antibodies were evaluated at three time points: preoperatively, 6 weeks postoperatively, and 3 months postoperatively. None of the 14 subjects exhibited antibodies to rhBMP-2. Two subjects exhibited positive antibody responses to bovine type I collagen at 6 weeks. Two of these remained positive at 3 months. No subjects were positive for antibodies to human type I collagen. All subjects with positive antibody responses were determined to have radiographic fusion at their last examination.

These pilot study results were very encouraging and confirmed the results from the previous preclinical and safety studies. The pilot trial provided the positive results that were necessary to enroll patients for a much larger clinical study. FDA approval to begin enrolling patients was obtained in July 1998, with the first patient enrolled in August of the same year.

Figure 6-4

A, INFUSE® Bone Graft and **B,** autograft patient CT scans from the pilot study at 6, 12, and 24 months postoperatively.

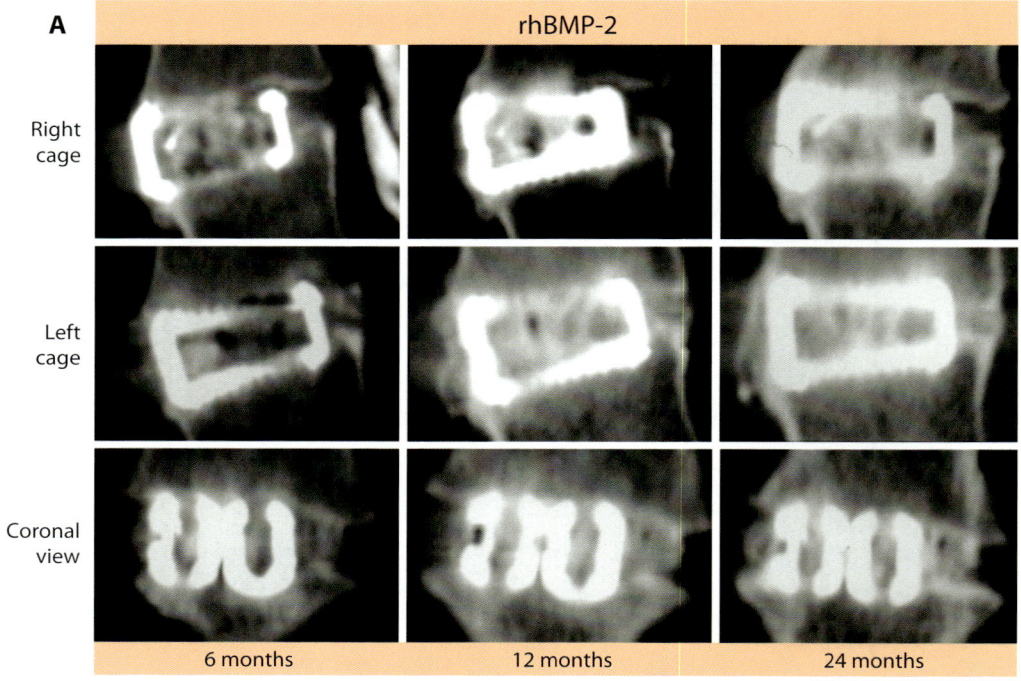

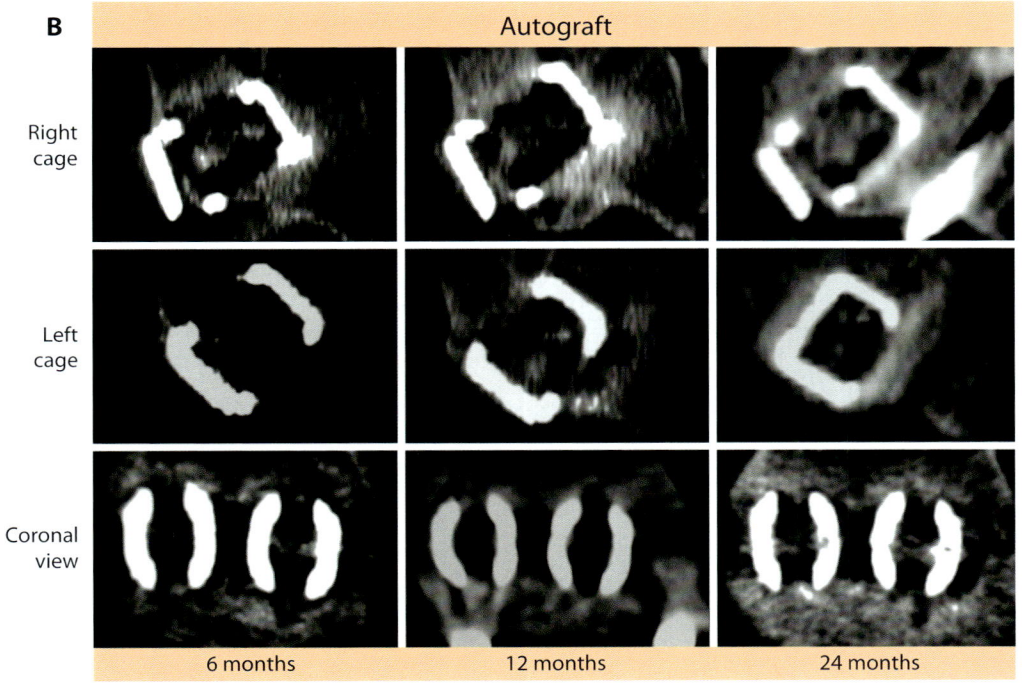

INFUSE® Bone Graft/LT-CAGE® Lumbar Tapered Fusion Device Pivotal Clinical Study Results

In a prospective, randomized IDE clinical study, 279 patients had surgery at 16 investigational sites.[3] All patients underwent a single-level anterior lumbar interbody fusion using two LT-CAGE® Devices. Patients were randomly assigned to one of two groups: The investigational group received INFUSE® Bone Graft (1.5 mg/cc rhBMP-2/ACS), and the control group received autologous iliac crest bone graft. Preoperatively, all patients had symptomatic, single-level, degenerative lumbar disc disease and symptoms of disabling low back and/or leg pain of a least 6 months' duration that had not responded to nonoperative treatments. The two treatment groups were very similar demographically. There were no statistically significant differences for any of the patient variables (Table 6-1).

Patient assessments were completed preoperatively, during hospitalization, and postoperatively at 6 weeks and at 3, 6, 12, and 24 months. Clinical outcomes were assessed using neurologic status, work status, patient satisfaction, the Oswestry Low Back Pain Disability Questionnaire, and back, leg and graft site pain questionnaires. Radiographic and CT scans were used to evaluate fusion at 6, 12, and 24 months after surgery (see the box on p. 129). Independent, blinded radiologists interpreted all radiographs and CT scans. At 6, 12, and 24 months after surgery, there was good agreement among the radiologists reviewing the scans (>98%). Fusion success was based on both clinical symptoms and radiographic findings. Patients who had secondary surgeries because of persistent low back symptoms and clinically suspected nonunions were considered as having failed fusion and were classified as failures in all fusion calculations, regardless of their independent radiologic assessment.

All patients underwent the ALIF procedure through an open approach. In the investigational group, each cage was filled with INFUSE® Bone Graft. No autogenous bone grafts or local reaming were used in this group. The control group received morselized autogenous iliac crest graft placed within the cages. The mean operative time in the control group was

Table 6-1

Demographic Data From INFUSE® Bone Graft/LT-CAGE® Device Pivotal Study

	Control	INFUSE® Bone Graft
Number	136	143
Age (yr)	42.3	43.3
Weight (lb)	181.1	179.1
Sex (male/female)	68/68	78/65
Workers' compensation (%)	34.6	32.9
Spinal litigation (%)	16.2	12.6
Tobacco use (%)	36.0	32.9
History of previous surgeries	40.4	37.8
Preoperative work status (%)	36.8	47.6

Criteria Used to Define Fusion on Radiographs and CT Scans

- Continuous bridging trabecular bone growth connecting the vertebral bodies on CT scan
- Translation of ≤3 mm
- Angulation of <5 degrees on flexion-extension radiograph
- Absence of radiolucent lines covering >50% of either implant

significantly longer than in the INFUSE® Bone Graft group (Table 6-2). The average blood loss was also significantly more in the control as compared to the group treated with INFUSE® Bone Graft. Discharge from the hospital was based on the treating surgeon's standard criteria; therefore the average hospital stay was similar in both groups.

In the control group, 8 adverse events related to harvesting the iliac crest graft were identified in 8 patients (5.9%). None required an additional surgery. The level of postoperative pain and morbidity associated with the iliac crest graft harvesting was measured using numeric rating scales for pain intensity and duration (Fig. 6-5). At discharge, all of the control patients experienced donor site hip pain with a mean score of 12.7 points out of 20 points. At 24 months after surgery, nearly one third of the control patients (32%) still experienced donor site hip pain.

The Oswestry Questionnaire (scale 0 to 100) was administered preoperatively and at each postoperative visit. The mean overall Oswestry scores for both treatment groups were similar at each of the time periods. At all postoperative visits, a statistical improvement in the average scores was observed for both treatment groups as compared with their preoperative scores (Fig. 6-6). The mean preoperative Oswestry score was 55.1 for the control group and 53.7 for the INFUSE® Bone Graft treatment group. At 24 months, the mean improvement in the Oswestry scores was 29.5 points

Table 6-2

Comparison of Surgical Data Between Groups

	Control	INFUSE® Bone Graft
Operative time (hr)	2.0	1.6
Blood loss (ml)	153.1	109.8
Hospital stay (days)	3.3	3.1

Figure 6-5

Percentage of autograft patients with donor site hip pain.

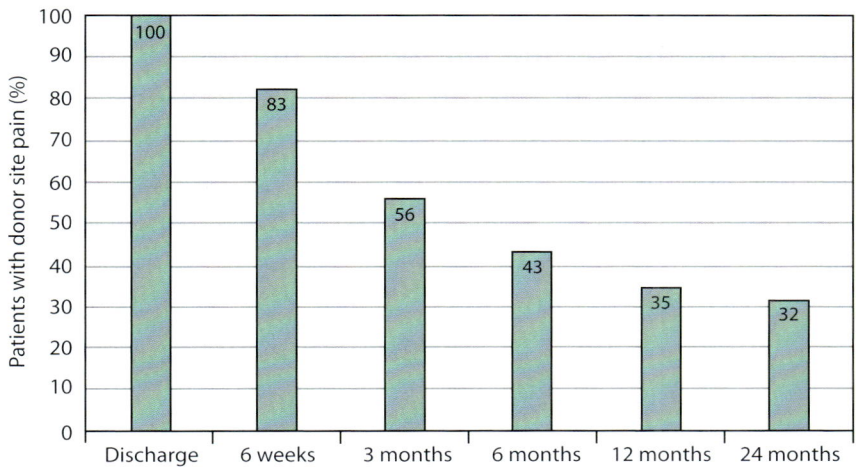

Figure 6-6

Comparison of the average Oswestry scores between groups. At 24 months the mean improvement in Oswestry score was 29.0 points for the INFUSE® Bone Graft group and 29.5 points for the autograft group.

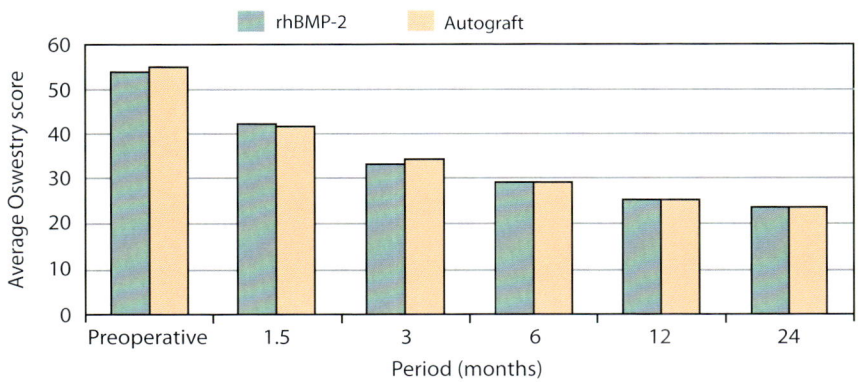

in the control group and 29.0 points in the INFUSE® Bone Graft treatment group (representing a 54% improvement for both groups).

Back pain intensity and duration were assessed using a 20-point numeric rating. A composite back pain score can be calculated by combining the numeric rating scores for the intensity and duration (Fig. 6-7). Leg pain was assessed in a similar manner using a numeric rating scale for both the intensity and duration symptoms. Outcomes were similar in both treatment groups (Fig. 6-8).

Fusion status of the study patients was evaluated on plain radiographs and CT scans. Patients who had secondary posterior stabilization procedures were reported as failed fusions without consideration of their radiographic findings. Results using this assessment method are shown in Fig. 6-9. Fusion rates decreased over time for two reasons: Radiolucencies from

Figure 6-7

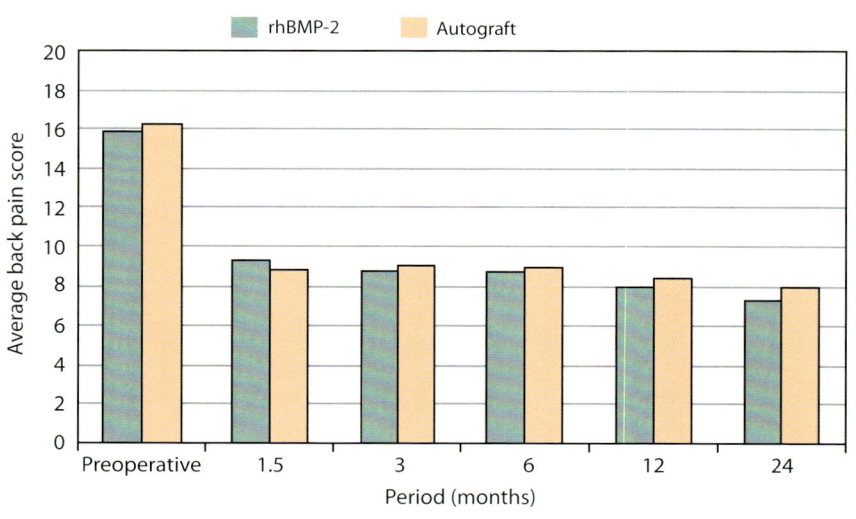

Comparison of average low back pain scores between groups.

Figure 6-8

Comparison of average leg pain scores between groups.

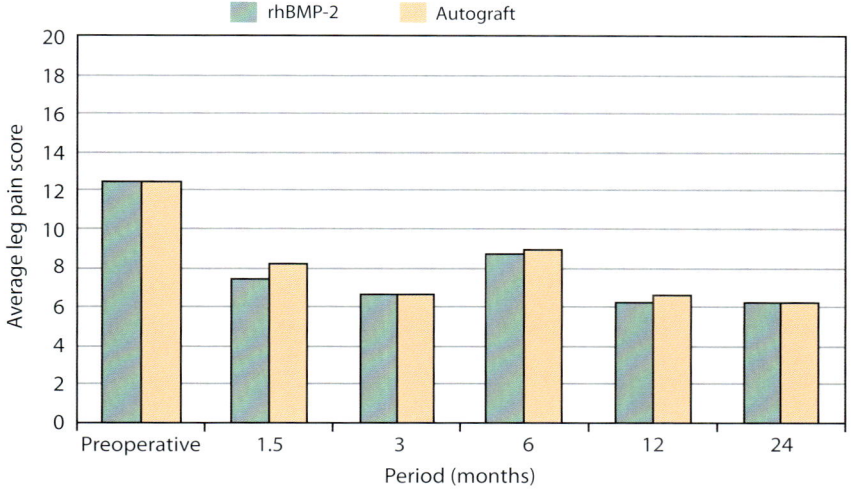

 Figure 6-9

Comparison of fusion rates between groups.

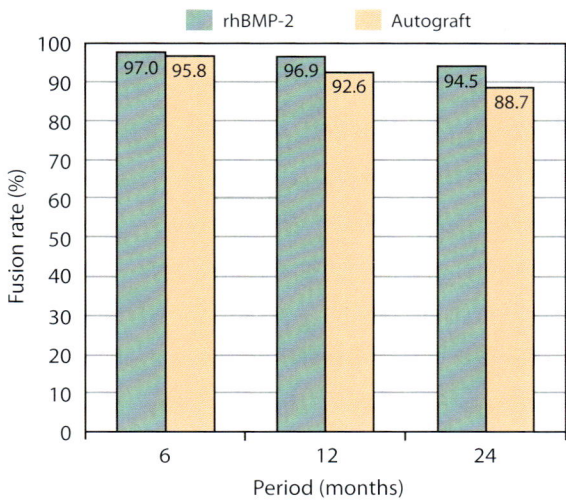

micromotion at the interface were identified and patients with persistent low back symptoms that warranted additional posterior stabilization surgery were classified as having a failed fusion. This is a very conservative and critical approach to assessing fusion, based on the IDE criteria (see box on p. 129).

The presence of antibodies to rhBMP-2 and bovine and human type I collagen was assessed preoperatively and at 3 months after surgery. Immune response to the INFUSE® Bone Graft components was evaluated in 349 investigational patients and 183 control patients receiving lumbar interbody fusions in multiple clinical trials. Results were similar between the two treatment groups (Table 6-3). No patients developed antibodies to human type I collagen. An evaluation was performed on the impact of a positive antibody response on overall success and fusion success. There was very little difference in overall and individual success when antibody status was taken into consideration. Moreover, the presence of antibodies to rhBMP-2 was not associated with immune-mediated adverse events

Table 6-3

Rates of Positive Antibody Response*

	Control (%)	INFUSE® Bone Graft (%)
rhBMP-2 antibody	0.8	0.7
Bovine type I collagen antibody	14.2	18.1
Human type I collagen antibody	0	0

*From package insert.

such as allergic reactions. The neutralizing capacity of antibodies to rhBMP-2 is not known.

This study demonstrated that treatment of DDD with the INFUSE® Bone Graft/LT-CAGE® Lumbar Tapered Fusion Device was as effective as the control treatment. The INFUSE® Bone Graft/LT-CAGE® Device was able to achieve comparable clinical performance while avoiding the necessity of an iliac crest graft harvest and its associated pain.

Metal constructs have been very successful in bringing spinal fusion technology a large step forward. Biotechnology, by ushering in rhBMP-2, provided a leap in spinal fusion technology that has allowed unprecedented control of the biologic aspect of bone formation. INFUSE® Bone Graft and the LT-CAGE® Lumbar Tapered Fusion Device form a pivotal combination of metal and biological technology for the spine.

Frequently Asked Questions

How were the clinical results studied?

The clinical results were evaluated using several methods of data analysis, including the Oswestry Low Back Pain Disability Questionnaire, Short Form SF-36, and neurologic status, work status, and back and leg pain questionnaires. CT scans and radiographs were also used to assess bone fusion, and findings were interpreted by two independent radiologists by blinded method (a third radiologist was consulted in the event of conflicting results).

Is there additional clinical experience with INFUSE® Bone Graft or rhBMP-2?

Medtronic Sofamor Danek has sponsored multiple FDA-approved multicenter clinical investigations of rhBMP-2 involving spine fusion (Fig. 6-10). These studies include the evaluation of applications for anterior and posterior lumbar interbody fusions, cervical fusions, and posterolateral fusions using a variety of different implants and instrumentation. The ALIF clinical studies described in this chapter were instrumental in gaining FDA approval of the INFUSE® Bone Graft/Interbody Fusion Device in 2002. Eventually, the other clinical trials will establish the clinical efficacy of rhBMP-2 in future FDA approvals. For now, these are considered investigational devices limited by U.S. law to investigational use only. This limitation pertains to unapproved, off-label use of INFUSE® Bone Graft. Medtronic Sofamor Danek does not recommend the use of its products in any manner other than those detailed in the package insert (see Fig. 6-1).

The location and extent of bone formation resulting from the use of osteoinductive proteins like rhBMP-2 depends on the placement of the implant, the carrier, and its proximity to bleeding bone.

The protocols for all of the rhBMP-2 clinical trials supported by Medtronic Sofamor Danek include radiographic analyses based on both plain radiographs and CT scans to provide a detailed assessment of new bone formation.

With the availability of INFUSE® Bone Graft, it will be important for spine surgeons to consider both mechanical and biologic factors, and it may be advantageous for surgeons to slightly modify surgical techniques to minimize potential concerns for certain selected procedures (such as posterior interbody fusions).

Figure 6-10

Multicenter clinical trials are being conducted to investigate the use of rhBMP-2 as an alternative to iliac crest autograft for spinal fusion applications. Contact Medtronic Sofamor Danek, Office of Medical Affairs for more information (1-800-876-3133). Subject to U.S. notice of availability.

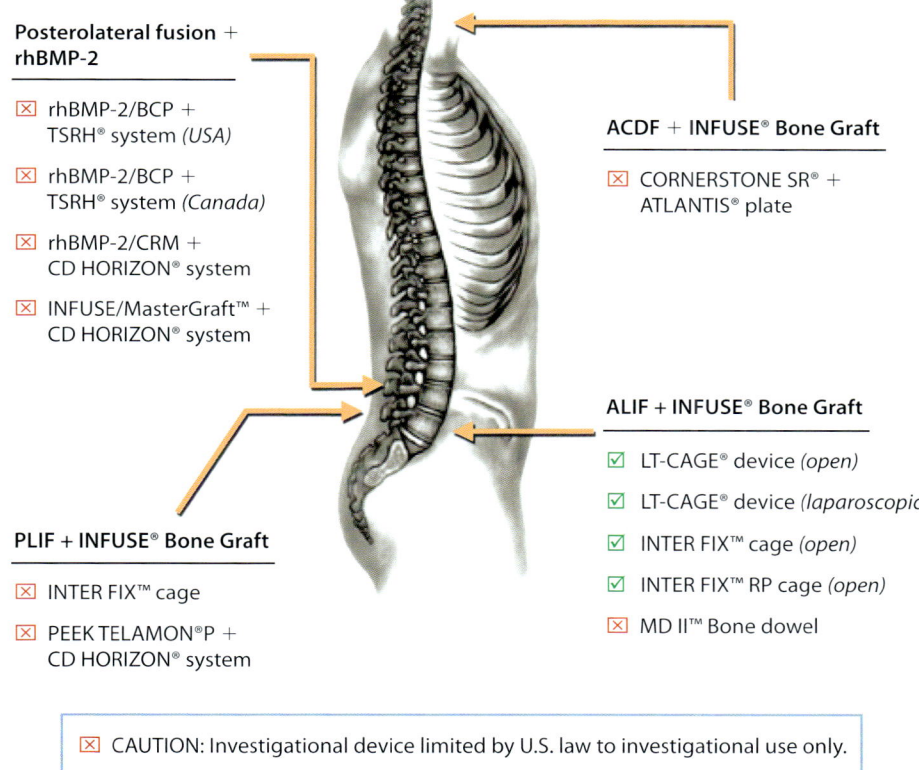

Posterolateral fusion + rhBMP-2
- ☒ rhBMP-2/BCP + TSRH® system *(USA)*
- ☒ rhBMP-2/BCP + TSRH® system *(Canada)*
- ☒ rhBMP-2/CRM + CD HORIZON® system
- ☒ INFUSE/MasterGraft™ + CD HORIZON® system

ACDF + INFUSE® Bone Graft
- ☒ CORNERSTONE SR® + ATLANTIS® plate

ALIF + INFUSE® Bone Graft
- ☑ LT-CAGE® device *(open)*
- ☑ LT-CAGE® device *(laparoscopic)*
- ☑ INTER FIX™ cage *(open)*
- ☑ INTER FIX™ RP cage *(open)*
- ☒ MD II™ Bone dowel

PLIF + INFUSE® Bone Graft
- ☒ INTER FIX™ cage
- ☒ PEEK TELAMON®P + CD HORIZON® system

☒ CAUTION: Investigational device limited by U.S. law to investigational use only.

When anterior cervical spinal fusions were performed using the INFUSE® Bone Graft component, some cases of edema have been reported within the first postoperative week. In some of these cases this swelling has been severe enough to produce airway compromise, sometimes requiring emergency surgery.

How was symptomatic lumbar degenerative disc disease determined?

The patients were evaluated based on instability, osteophyte formation, decreased disc height, thickening of ligamentous tissue, disc herniation, and facet joint degeneration.

REFERENCES

1. Zdeblick TA, Boden SD, Sandhu HS. The clinical use of rhBMP-2 in interbody fusion cages. Presented at the Thirteenth Annual Meeting of the North American Spine Society, San Francisco, Calif, 1998.
2. Boden SD, Zdeblick TA, Sandhu HS, et al. The use of rhBMP-2 in interbody fusion cages. Definitive evidence of osteoinduction in humans: A preliminary report. Spine 25:376-381, 2000.
3. Burkus JK, Gornet MF, Dickman CA, et al. Anterior lumbar interbody fusion using rhBMP-2 with tapered interbody cages. J Spinal Disord Tech 15:337-349, 2002.

INDEX

A

Absorbable collagen sponge; *see* Collagen sponge, absorbable
Absorption of rhBMP-2, 53
Achilles tendon, collagen sponge from, 69
ACS; *see* Collagen sponge, absorbable
Acute toxicity study, 45-47
Allograft bone dowel, 93-99
American Society for Testing and Materials (ASTM), 10
Anatomic location, healing rate of, 90-92
Antibody
    to absorbable collagen sponge, 82
    in INFUSE® Bone Graft study, 125, 134
Assay
    osteoinductivity, 10-11
    rat ectopic bone, 10
Autograft
    histologic assessment of, 92-96
    iliac crest, rhBMP-2/ACS versus, 100-101
    local, limitations of, 5
Autoimmune reaction to collagen sponge, 82
Autologous bone graft, 24
    rhBMP-2 as enhancer for, 106-108

B

Binding of rhBMP-2 with absorbable collagen sponge, 70-73
Biocompatibility test, 76, 77
Biodistribution of rhBMP-2, 52-55
Biphasic calcium phosphate, 108-109
Bleeding bone, 91, 114
Blood loss during surgery, 130
BMP; *see* Bone morphogenetic protein
BMP-2, 28-30, 32-33
BMPRI, 32
BMPRIIB, 32
Bone
    bleeding, 91, 114
    components of, 25
    local autograft versus iliac crest, 5
    repair of, 27-33
Bone assay, rat ectopic, 10
Bone dowel, allograft, 93-99
Bone formation
    BMP-2 in, 28-30, 32-33
    rhBMP-2/ACS-induced, 79-80, 83
Bone graft enhancer, 106-108
Bone graft extender, 5-8
Bone graft replacement
    burden of proof for, 14-15
    challenges of, 3-4
    need for, 2
    options for, 5-8
    requirements for, 2-3
Bone growth, 114
Bone morphogenetic protein
    autograft bone versus, 16
    binding to mesenchymal stem cells, 32
    definition of, 26
    in demineralized bone matrix, 19
    demineralized bone matrix versus, 12-13
    discovery of, 24-25
    familiarity with, 16
    frequently asked questions about, 37-38
    Humanitarian Device Exemptions regulation and, 19-20
    induction of new bone by, 10
    in INFUSE® Bone Graft versus OP-1® Putty, 17-18, 19
    other growth factors versus, 34-35
    products containing, 16-17
    recombinant human; *see* rhBMP-2
    roles of, 27-33

Bone morphogenetic protein—cont'd
    sources of, 35-37
    species-specific healing rates for, 90-92
    types of, 26-27
Bovine collagen, 69
    antibodies to, 125, 134
Bovine spongiform encephalitis, 81
Bulking agent, 108-109
Burden of proof for fusion graft replacement, 14-15

C

C26 cell, 30
Cage, metal, 93-99
Cancer, rhBMP-2 study of, 56-57
Canine study
    of graft enhancer, 106
    of mandibular/maxillofacial inlay, 73-76
    of rhBMP-2, 46-47, 48-49
    of spinal tissue effects, 110-114
Carcinogenicity study, 56-57, 62-63
Carrier
    absorbable collagen sponge as, 68-85; see also Collagen sponge, absorbable
    amount of rhBMP-2 delivered in, 88, 89
    for interbody fusion, 94
    for rhBMP-2, 58-61
Cell
    mesenchymal, 28
    migration of, 28-30
    osteoprogenitor, 2
Cell line assay for osteoinductivity, 10-11
Cell line study, tumor growth, 56-57
Chemotaxis, 28, 29
Chronic toxicity study of rhBMP-2/ACS, 73-76
Clinical efficacy study; see INFUSE® Bone Graft/LT-CAGE® Lumbar Tapered Fusion Device
Collagen, antibodies to, 125, 134
Collagen sponge, absorbable
    antibodies and, 82
    binding to rhBMP-2, 70-73
    biocompatibility studies of, 76, 77
    biodistribution studies of, 77-78
    clinical history of, 80
    description of, 69
    frequently asked questions about, 80-83
    in INFUSE® Bone Graft, 120
    limitations of, for posterolateral fusion, 101-105
    quality of bone formed, 83
    resorption rate of, 82
    retained in body, 81
    soaking time for, 80
    timing of bone formation with, 79-80
    viral safety of, 81
Compression-resistant matrix, 109
Computed tomography (CT)
    for assessment of INFUSE® Bone Graft, 124
    criteria for defining fusion, 129
    to evaluate spinal fusion, 93
    in INFUSE® Bone Graft study, 126-127
    sensitivity of, to mature bone, 83
Concentration
    of bone morphogenetic protein, species-specific, 90
    of rhBMP-2, 88, 89
Criteria
    for defining fusion, 129
    for fusion graft replacement, 14-15
Culture medium for rhBMP-2, 44

D

Degenerative disc disease, 124
Demineralization, osteoinductive potential of, 25
Demineralized bone matrix, 12-13, 18
Demographic data from INFUSE® Bone Graft/LT-CAGE® Lumbar Tapered Fusion Device study, 129
Dibotermin alfa, 7-8
Disability questionnaire, low back pain, 125, 130-132
Discovery of bone morphogenetic protein, 24-25
Dowel, allograft bone, 93-99
Dura, 114

E

Ectopic rat model, 10
    bone formation in, 28
Endochondral bone, formation of, 29
Endplate, bleeding, 91

Enhancer, graft, 106-108
Excretion of rhBMP-2, 54, 62
Extender, bone graft, 5-8
Extract, 35

F

FDA approval for INFUSE® Bone Graft/Interbody Fusion Device, 136
Fetal study, 50-52, 63-64
Formation of bone, 27-33
Fusion, spinal
  challenges of, 3-4
  determination of dosage and concentration for, 88, 89
  evaluation techniques for, 92-93
  frequently asked questions about, 114-115
  graft requirements for, 2-3
  iliac crest autograft in, 100-101
  limitations of carrier in, 101-105
  metal cages versus allograft bone dowels for, 93-99
  posterolateral, 108-109
    collagen sponge carrier in, 101-105
    interbody fusion versus, 91
  radiographic and CT criteria for, 129
  species-specific healing rates and, 90-92
  spinal tissue effects and, 110-114

G

Graft; see also Bone graft entries
  extender of, 5-8
  xenograft as source of BMP, 36
Graft enhancer, potential, 106-108
Graft replacement; see Bone graft replacement
Granule, HA/TCP, 109
Growth factor, 34-35
  transforming growth factor-β, 12, 26
Growth medium for rhBMP-2 production, 37

H

HA/TCP granule, 109
Healing
  bone, 3, 24
  species-specific rates for, 90-92
Histologic study
  in interbody fusion evaluation, 95, 96
  radiography versus, 92

Human type I collagen, antibodies to, 125, 134
Humanitarian Device Exemption (HDE), 19-21
Humanitarian Use Device
  marketing of, 19
  off-label use of, 20
Hydroxyapatite, 109

I

Identification of rhBMP-2, 42
Iliac crest autograft
  as gold standard, 24
  rhBMP-2/ACS versus, 100-101
Iliac crest bone
  local autograft bone versus, 5
  rationale for using, 4
Implant model, rat subcutaneous, 6, 7
InductOs, 121
INFUSE® Bone Graft
  bone morphogenetic protein in, 16
  dosage of, 114
  production of, 62
  properties of, 7-8
INFUSE® Bone Graft/Interbody Fusion Device, FDA approval of, 136
INFUSE® Bone Graft/LT-CAGE® Lumbar Tapered Fusion Device, 117-138
  characteristics of, 120-121
  frequently asked questions about, 135-138
  graft volume guide for, 123
  indications and contraindications for, 119
  kit components, 122
  pilot study results of, 121-127
  pivotal clinical study results with, 128-135
  scans of, 126-127
Institutional Review Board, 20
Interbody fusion
  with metal cages and allograft bone dowels, 93-99
  posterolateral fusion versus, 91
Investigational Device Exemption trial, 121, 123

L

Laminectomy, 112
Local autograft bone, limitations of, 5
Low back pain disability questionnaire, 125, 130-132

M

Matrix, compression-resistant, 109
Medium, culture, for rhBMP-2, 44
Medtronic Sofamor Danek, 62, 121, 136
Mesenchymal cell, 28
    bone morphogenetic protein binding to, 32
    differentiation of, 31
Metabolism, of rhBMP-2, 52-55
Metal cage, 93-99
Migration, cell, 28-30
Mitogenic factor, 30
Monkey study of metal cages versus allograft bone dowels, 99
Morphogenetic protein, bone; *see* Bone morphogenetic protein
Multipotent cell line, 30

O

Off-label use of Humanitarian Device Exemption product, 20
OP-1® Putty, 17-18, 19
Osteoblast, 32-33
Osteoinductivity, 6-8
    assays for, 10-11
    of bone morphogenetic protein, 27-28
    importance of, 9
    osteoconductivity versus, 8-9
Osteoprogenitor cell, 2
Oswestry Low Back Pain Disability Questionnaire, 125, 130-132

P

Perinatal study of rhBMP-2, 52
Pharmacokinetic study
    of BMP-2, 55
    of rhBMP-2/ACS, 78
Platelet-rich plasma, 34-35
Posterolateral fusion
    bulking agents in, 108-109
    collagen sponge carrier in, 101-105
    interbody fusion versus, 91
Preclinical efficacy study of rhBMP-2, 87-116
    dosage and concentration for, 88, 89
    frequently asked questions about, 114-115
    fusion evaluation in, 92-93
    as graft enhancer, 106-108
    iliac crest autograft compared with, 100-101
    limitations of carrier in, 101-105
    with metal cages and allograft bone dowels, 93-99
    posterolateral, 108-109
    species-specific healing rates and, 90-92
    of spinal tissue effects, 110-114
    summary of, 102-103
Protein, bone morphogenetic; *see* Bone morphogenetic protein

Q

Questionnaire, low back pain disability, 125, 130-132

R

Rabbit, posterolateral fusion in, 104
Radiographic evaluation
    criteria for defining fusion, 129
    histologic studies versus, 92
    of interbody fusion, 96
Rat ectopic bone assay
    of osteoinductivity, 10
    with platelet-rich plasma versus BMP-2, 34-35
Rat study
    of absorbable collagen sponge, 73-76
    of healing rate, 90
    of rhBMP-2, 45-46, 48
Rat subcutaneous implant model, 6, 7
Recombinant human bone morphogenetic protein; *see* rhBMP-2
Recombination process, 42-43
Repair, bone, bone morphogenetic protein in, 27-33
Reproductive study, 50-52
Research, 37
Resorption of absorbable collagen sponge, 82
Review, Institutional Review Board, 20
rhBMP-2, 7-8
    activation of, 38
    acute toxicity studies of, 45-47
    allograft bone dowels filled with, 93-99
    binding with absorbable collagen sponge, 70-73
    biodistribution and metabolism studies of, 52-55

carcinogenicity of, 56-57
carrier for, 58-61
characterization of, 38
clinical efficacy study of, 117-138
description of, 42-44
dose of, 88, 89
excretion of, 62
frequently asked questions about, 62-64
identification of, 42
preclinical efficacy study of, 87-116
reproductive effects studies of, 50-52
safety of, 45, 62
subchronic toxicity studies of, 48-50
rhBMP-2/ACS
   biocompatibility testing of, 76, 77
   biodistribution study of, 77-78
   CT assessment and, 83
   implantation site and, 83
   preparation instructions for, 88
   quality of bone formed with, 83
   safety of, 73-76
   volume of, 88

S
Safety
   of absorbable collagen sponge, 73
   of rhBMP-2, 45, 62
Sheep study, to evaluation spinal fusion, 92-93
Soaking of absorbable collagen sponge, 80
Species-specific rate
   of bone formation, 60
   of healing, 90-92
Spinal fusion; *see* Fusion, spinal
Sponge, absorbable collagen; *see* Collagen sponge, absorbable
Spongiform encephalitis, bovine, 81
Stability of absorbable collagen sponge, 81
Stem cell, mesenchymal, 28
Sterility of absorbable collagen sponge, 81
Stiffness, preclinical study of, 105
Strength, preclinical study of, 105
Subchronic toxicity study, 48-50
Subcutaneous implant model, rat, 6, 7
Swelling, postoperative, 75

T
Tendon, Achilles, 69
TGF-β; see Transforming growth factor-β
Timing, rhBMP-2/ACS-induced bone formation, 79-80
Titanium device, 136
Toxicity study
   of absorbable collagen sponge, 73-76
   of rhBMP-2, 45-50, 114
Transforming growth factor-β
   bone formation and, 12
   bone morphogenetic protein related to, 26
Transmissible spongiform encephalitis, 81
Tricalcium phosphate, 109
Trichloroacetic acid, in BMP-2 study, 54
Tumor growth, rhBMP-2 and, 56-57

U
Undifferentiated cell, mesenchymal stem cells as, 31
Urist, Dr. Marshall, 24-25

V
Viral safety of absorbable collagen sponge, 81

X
Xenograft as source of BMP, 36